Drug-Induced Osteonecrosis of the Jaws

How to Diagnose, Prevent, and Treat It

Drug-Induced Osteonecrosis of the Jaws

How to Diagnose, Prevent, and Treat It

Robert E. Marx, DDS, FACS

Professor of Surgery and Chief
Division of Oral and Maxillofacial Surgery
Miller School of Medicine
University of Miami
Miami, Florida

QUINTESSENCE PUBLISHING

Berlin | Chicago | Tokyo
Barcelona | London | Milan | Mexico City | Moscow | Paris | Prague | Seoul | Warsaw
Beijing | Istanbul | Sao Paulo | Zagreb

Library of Congress Cataloging-in-Publication Data

Names: Marx, Robert E., author.
Title: Drug-induced osteonecrosis of the jaws : how to diagnose, prevent, and treat it / Robert E. Marx.
Description: Batavia, IL : Quintessence Publishing Co, Inc, [2021] | Includes bibliographical references and index. | Summary: "Explores the science behind DIONJ before presenting the protocols for treating the disease in patients with osteoporosis and/or cancer. Special attention is paid to how to prevent DIONJ from developing in vulnerable sites and populations"-- Provided by publisher.
Identifiers: LCCN 2021029327 | ISBN 9781647240899 (paperback)
Subjects: MESH: Bisphosphonate-Associated Osteonecrosis of the Jaw | Diphosphonates--adverse effects | Bone Density Conservation Agents--adverse effects | Antineoplastic Agents--adverse effects
Classification: LCC RC931.O73 | NLM WU 140.5 | DDC 616.7/1606--dc23
LC record available at https://lccn.loc.gov/2021029327

A CIP record for this book is available from the British Library.
ISBN: 9781647240899

QUINTESSENCE PUBLISHING
USA

Quintessence Publishing Co, Inc
411 N Raddant Road
Batavia, IL 60510
www.quintpub.com

5 4 3 2 1

Editor: Leah Huffman
Design: Sue Zubek
Production: Angelina Schmelter

Printed in Croatia

Contents

Dedication *vi*
Preface *vii*

1 Understanding Drug-Induced Osteonecrosis of the Jaws *1*

2 Prevention and Management of DIONJ in Patients Treated for Osteopenia/Osteoporosis *21*

3 Prevention and Management of DIONJ in Cancer Patients Taking Drugs Known to Cause DIONJ *59*

Index *89*

Dedication

Indeed, a dog can be man's best friend. I have been blessed to have grown up with and lived my adult life with such dogs. Due to their shorter life span than ours, their love and loyalty too often fade with the years. To commemorate that love and loyalty as well as every lick in the face, I want to dedicate this book to them in the order that they were with me: Blackie, Teeka, Cinder, Cindy, Lillie, Lucky, Rusty, Odie, Bones, Ninja, Rocky, Tubby, and Libby and Copper, who are still with me and my wife.

Preface

Dead bone in the mouth, known as *drug-induced osteonecrosis of the jaws (DIONJ)*, is a problem that every dental and oral and maxillofacial surgeon faces. It is also a problem that every oncologist faces.

What was first recognized in 2003 and linked to bisphosphonates has been expanded to include RANK ligand inhibitors and antiangiogenic drugs. The numbers of DIONJ cases have accumulated into tens of thousands and have caused bone loss, infection, pain, and deformity in many individuals. DIONJ is a drug complication that has not gone away, nor is it likely to go away. Most of the responsibility in preventing and managing the complication of this medical drug therapy falls on the dental profession and its specialties.

This author has published two previous texts on DIONJ (2007 and 2011) identifying the biologic mechanism of bone necrosis, its pathophysiology, and suggestions on its management. This new text accepts and does not dwell on the known pathophysiology of DIONJ from each drug. Instead, it concentrates its attention on specific measures the clinician can practice to prevent DIONJ, to assess risk, to slow its progress, to prevent worsening it, and to resolve it when it does occur.

This text, with its case samples, outlines specific medical history questions to ask patients as well as specific caveats of the oral examination related to DIONJ identification and assessment. It also presents specific antibiotic protocols that have proven best in controlling secondary infection. A new and more useable staging system is introduced that will help the clinician in disease assessment and treatment planning.

For the osteoporosis/osteopenia patient, the effective use of drug holidays allows the dental and oral and maxillofacial surgeon to perform indicated procedures with greater safety. The newly discovered role of occlusion and occlusal trauma in initiating DIONJ has led to the before-unrecognized preventive value of occlusal adjustments, the splinting of teeth, and mouthguards.

It is hoped that this book will serve as a guide for each provider to lessen the impact of DIONJ on their patients while still maintaining the dental and reconstruction/rehabilitation services we are known to provide.

Chapter 1

Understanding Drug-Induced Osteonecrosis of the Jaws

What is now most accurately termed *drug-induced osteonecrosis of the jaws (DIONJ)*[1] came upon the dental scene in 2003.[2,3] Since then, there have been over 2,500 refereed articles published on it. Every specialty of dentistry has produced a position paper on it. Every drug company manufacturing one of the offending drugs has a warning in its advertising referring to "dental problems" or "jaw problems." And most every practicing dentist has seen one or more cases.

Although numerous other terms for DIONJ have been advanced, such as *medicine-related osteonecrosis of the jaws (MRONJ),*[4] *bisphosphonate-associated osteonecrosis of the jaws (BAONJ),*[5] and *chemo-osteonecrosis of the jaws (CONJ),*[6] among others, DIONJ is the most correct due to its identification of a cause-and-effect relationship, its acknowledgment that drugs other than bisphosphonates cause it, and because it is consistent with the term adopted by the World Health Organization and published by the American Medical Association ICD-10 code (M87.10).[1] Nevertheless, by any term, the dental profession has come to recognize the necrotic bone in either jaw as osteonecrosis caused by certain drugs.

How Do These Drugs Kill Jaw Bone?

The basic mechanism of the most common drugs known to cause DIONJ is that they are cellular poisons that affect bone remodeling and renewal. A few others cause DIONJ by affecting the blood supply to bone.

Bone is derived from osteoblasts, which secrete osteoid. These cells become entrapped in their mineralized matrix to become osteocytes, which have a life span of about 180 days. During this time, they secrete a protein called *osteoprotegerin,* which competes and inhibits RANK ligand (reactive activator of nuclear κB ligand).[7] Because RANK ligand is a natural activator of osteoclasts, this process resists bone resorption and maintains the bone during the 180-day life span of the osteocyte.

The basic mechanism of the most common drugs known to cause DIONJ is that they are cellular poisons that affect bone remodeling and renewal.

When the osteocyte ages or dies off at the end of its life span or from injury, its production of osteoprotegerin ceases, allowing RANK ligand to stimulate osteoclasts to resorb old dysfunctional bone, injured bone, or dead bone. This process is an evolutionary homeostatic process that maintains our skeletons in a healthy state, with bone capable of withstanding loads with proper elasticity and integrity.

Therefore, the clinician should understand that the mandible and the maxilla are not static and are turning over daily. In fact, the alveolar bone of the jaws turns over at a rate that is 10 times faster than that of long bones,[8] which is why DIONJ always begins in the alveolar bone. As such, the most vulnerable areas of the jaws are those areas where bone turnover is the greatest—ie, extraction sockets, the posterior lingual areas around mandibular molars, the maxillary alveolus and floor of the sinus above the maxillary molars, areas of alveolar bone surgery, areas of chronic occlusal overloading, and the surface of tori.[9]

The alveolar bone of the jaws turns over at a rate that is 10 times faster than that of long bones,[8] which is why DIONJ always begins in the alveolar bone.

Femur fractures

This understanding of bone turnover and bone remodeling also predicted the midshaft femur fractures resulting from osteoporosis drugs first reported in 2008 and now recognized frequently by orthopedic surgeons.[10,11] This complication of DIONJ-causing drugs is now warned about by the drug companies.

The femur is the longest bone in the human skeleton. As we walk or run, we plant our feet so that the tibia/fibula and joints absorb the compressive forces. However, the femur flexes somewhat at its midshaft during this process as the knee bends. This creates an increased demand for bone remodeling and renewal in the midshaft areas, which after long-term use from many of the DIONJ-causing drugs results in a unique midshaft fracture due to the brittleness of the old unrenewed bone in that location (Fig 1-1).

Risk Factors for DIONJ

Unfortunately, drug companies and most position papers have published related "risk factors" that are not really risk factors for DIONJ at all. Publications have claimed that obesity or smoking,[12] anemia,[13] diabetes,[14] and many other common human habits and maladies cause DIONJ; however, these things do not actually cause osteonecrosis unless the individual has also been taking one of the drugs known to cause osteonecrosis. These are not risk factors by themselves. Therefore, the clinician examining or treating patients taking drugs that have

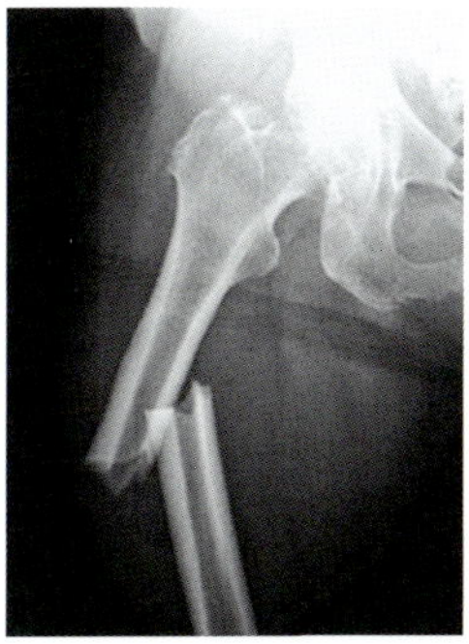

FIG 1-1 Atypical fracture of the femur caused by extended use of alendronate (Fosamax).

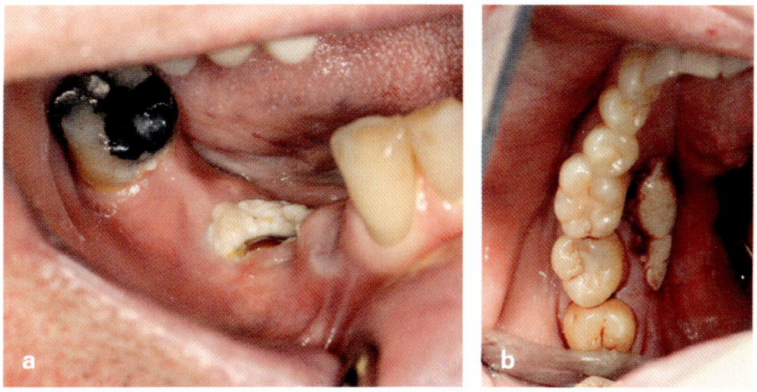

FIG 1-2 *(a)* DIONJ from alendronate in a patient treated for osteopenia. *(b)* DIONJ from denosumab in a patient treated for osteoporosis.

been known to cause DIONJ should keep in mind the seven critical aspects of risk described in the next section.

The drug itself

The only risk factor for DIONJ is the drug itself. The degree of the risk is related to the potency of the drug, the dose of the drug, the frequency that it is taken, the length of time the individual has taken the drug, its mechanism of action, and when the last dose was taken.

> The only risk factor for DIONJ is the drug itself.

1. Potency

The potency of oral bisphosphonates taken for osteoporosis is well known and is determined relative to the first bisphosphonate introduced: etidronate. Relating the potency of etidronate as 1, tiludronate is 50 times as potent, risedronate and ibandronate 1,000 times as potent, and alendronate 5,000 times as potent. The potency for subcutaneous denosumab, a RANK ligand inhibitor for osteoporosis, is not known as compared to bisphosphonates. However, from its mechanism of action and its track record of DIONJ, it is at least as potent as alendronate when prescribed for osteoporosis and even more potent than zoledronate when administered for cancer patients. In fact, alendronate and denosumab are responsible for over 97% of DIONJ cases in the noncancer patient treated for osteopenia/osteoporosis (Fig 1-2 and Table 1-1).

Table 1-1 Percentage of DIONJ cases in noncancer patients caused by various osteoporosis drugs (N = 211)

Drug	Dosage	N	%
Alendronate	70 mg per week	129	61%
Denosumab	60 mg every 6 months	76	36%
Risedronate	35 mg per week	4	2%
Ibandronate	150 mg per month	2	1%
Raloxifene	NA	0	0%
rhPTH 1-34	NA	0	0%
rhPTH 1-80	NA	0	0%
Vitamin D + calcium	NA	0	0%

This twofold higher dose underscores the danger of alendronate as a major risk factor for DIONJ.

2. Dose and frequency

While the dose of oral risedronate is 35 mg/week and the dose of oral ibandronate is 150 mg/month, which averages out to be 35 mg/week, the dose of oral alendronate is 70 mg/week. This twofold higher dose underscores the danger of alendronate as a major risk factor for DIONJ. Denosumab for the osteopenia/osteoporosis patient is a fixed dose of 60 mg administered subcutaneously every 6 months (see Table 1-1).

3. Half-life

One of the major distinctions between bisphosphonates and denosumab is their half-life in bone. All bisphosphonates become irreversibly bound to the mineral matrix in bone with a half-life of 11.2 years.[15] The affinity of bisphosphonates for bone is so great that when an osteoclast dies from ingesting a bisphosphonate and bursts, it releases the bisphosphonate. The bisphosphonate molecules are then rapidly reincorporated into adjacent bone. It is this cumulative buildup of bisphosphonate molecules in the more actively turning over alveolar bone that causes DIONJ from these drugs and targets the jaws.[9]

Denosumab does not become bound to bone and has a half-life of only 26 days.[16] However, its high potency and therefore its equal risk of causing DIONJ compared to alendronate is due to its mechanism of action affecting the very development of osteoclasts in the bone marrow.[17]

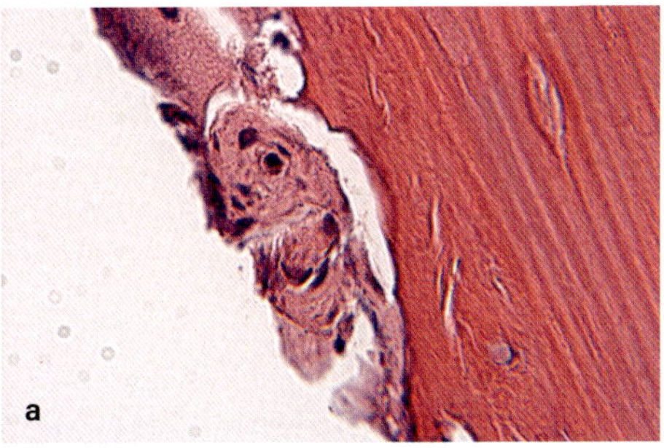
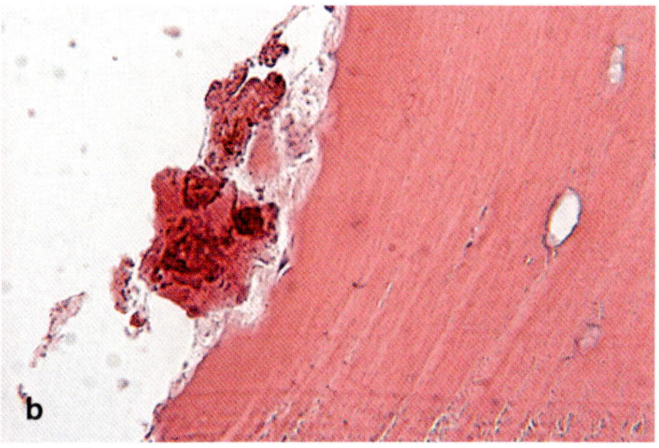
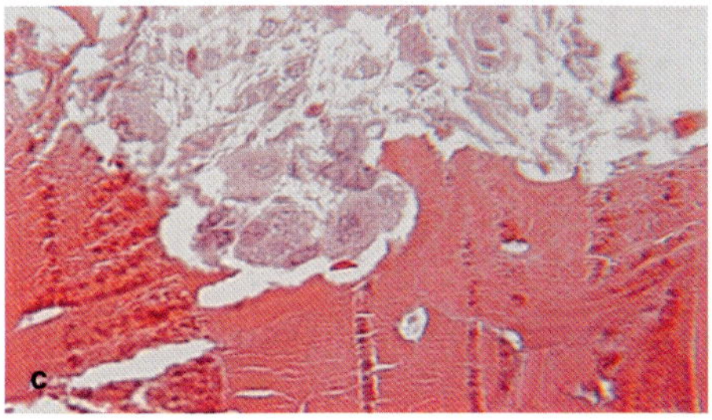

FIG 1-3 *(a)* Osteoclast resorbing bisphosphonate-loaded bone showing disruption of nuclei as a sign of early toxicity. *(b)* Pale and ballooned osteoclasts after ingesting a bisphosphonate during bone resorption before bursting. *(c)* Pale and ballooned osteoclasts with shrunken remnants of osteoclasts that have burst.

4. Mechanism of action

All bisphosphonates are cellular poisons that inhibit the cytoplasmic enzyme farnesyl synthetase required by nearly every cell.[18] The reason why osteoclasts are more greatly affected is that they ingest a high concentration of the bisphosphonate that accumulates into bone as they go about resorbing it. Essentially, the osteoclast is singled out because it is the cell that comes into contact with the greatest concentration of a bisphosphonate, and the jaws are singled out because of their constant need for osteoclast-mediated bone turnover due to occlusion and denture wearing. Other less frequent but noted complications from bisphosphonates such as esophagitis[19] and renal tubular necrosis[20] are also due to these tissues coming into contact with a greater concentration of bisphosphonates than other tissues.

Nevertheless, bisphosphonates' main toxicity is focused on the adult osteoclast as it resorbs bone that has accumulated a high concentration of bisphosphonate, with much less effect on developing osteoclasts in the bone marrow or circulating osteoclasts (Fig 1-3). That is, the main driving force of bisphosphonate toxicity is its half-life in bone and its accumulation from continuous dosing due to its irreversible biding to the mineral matrix of bone.[21,22]

The mechanism of action of denosumab in DIONJ is its inhibition of RANK ligand[23] (Fig 1-4a). However, RANK ligand is not only required to stimulate the adult osteoclast to resorb bone but is also required in nearly every maturation step of the osteoclast from the mononuclear bone marrow osteoclast precursor

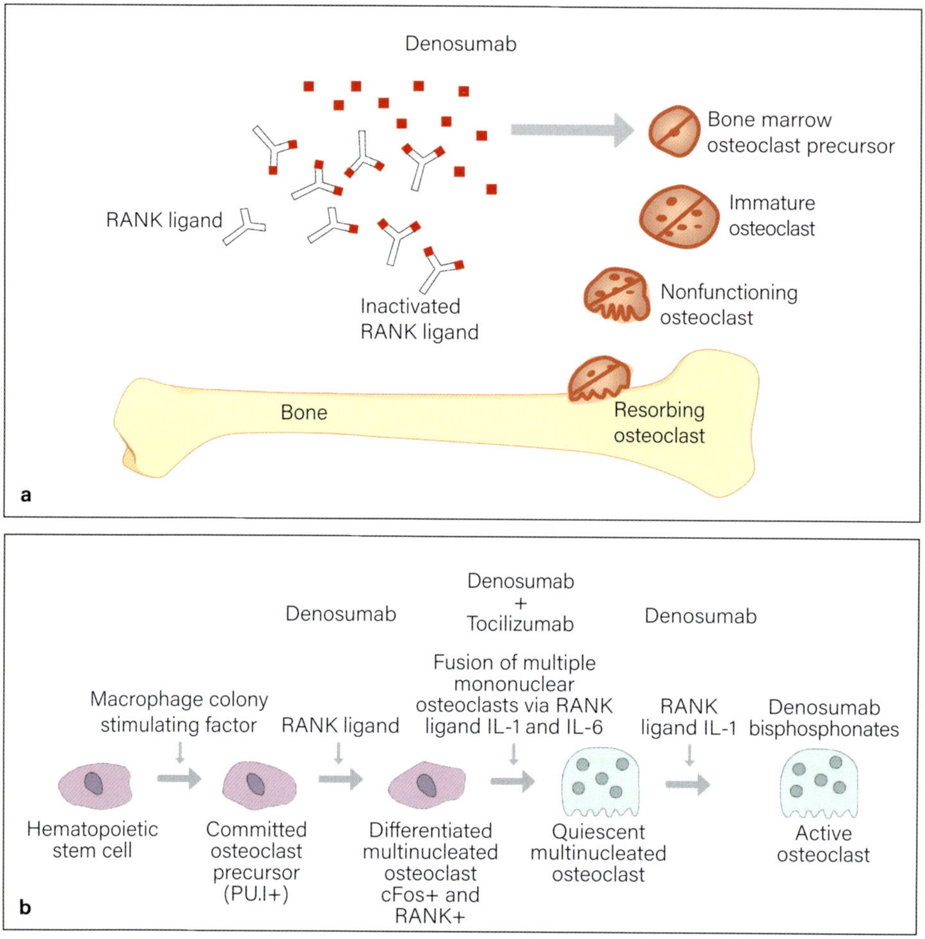

FIG 1-4 *(a)* Denosumab's inhibition of RANK ligand affects the mononuclear osteoclast precursors in the bone marrow, the developing osteoclasts in the bone marrow, the maturing osteoclasts, and the adult multinucleated osteoclasts. *(b)* Because RANK ligand is required in most phases of osteoclast development and maturity, RANK ligand inhibitors like denosumab have a profound negative effect on bone remodeling and renewal.

Table 1-2 Dosing risks of DIONJ after exposure to osteoporosis drugs

Drug	Risk begins	Mean dose for DIONJ
Oral alendronate (70 mg)	104th dose	240 doses
Intravenous zoledronate (4 or 5 mg)	4th dose	9 doses
Subcutaneous denosumab (60 mg every 6 mos)	4th dose	8 doses
Subcutaneous denosumab (120 mg/mo)	2nd dose	3 doses

to the multinucleated functioning osteoclast[9,24] (Fig 1-4b). It is this potent effect on the developing and circulating osteoclasts as well as the adult osteoclasts that make denosumab (60 mg every 6 months) a significant risk factor for DIONJ in the osteopenia/osteoporosis patient and an even greater risk factor when it is administered at 120 mg/month for cancer patients.

5. Length of time of drug use

Certainly the length of time the drug has been used relates to an increased risk. With bisphosphonate use, this increased risk comes from the accumulation of bisphosphonate molecules in bone over the time in which it has been taken due to its long half-life in bone. For denosumab, which has a short half-life of just 26 days, this increased risk relates to its multifocal inhibitory effects on developing osteoclasts in the bone marrow, the circulating osteoclasts in blood, and the adult osteoclast trying to resorb bone, thereby depleting the osteoclast population and reserves.

6. Route of administration

Bisphosphonates in the treatment of osteopenia/osteoporosis are mostly prescribed as oral drugs. However, the intravenous (IV) drug zoledronate, which is mostly used for cancer patients with bone metastasis, is also used for osteoporosis at a different dose and frequency, that is, 5 mg IV once per year. Whether for the treatment of osteopenia/osteoporosis (60 mg every 6 months) or cancer metastasis (120 mg/month), denosumab is always administered subcutaneously.

The difference between an oral and IV bisphosphonate is significant. An ingested oral bisphosphonate is poorly absorbed (ie, 0.68% in the gut). Therefore, there is a gradual accumulation of the oral bisphosphonate in bone. From the experience of the author, one must take an oral bisphosphonate for 2 years (104 doses) to begin to develop a risk for DIONJ, with the risk increasing with subsequent doses beyond that (Table 1-2). On the other hand, with IV zoledronate for either osteoporosis at 5 mg/year or for cancer at 4 mg/month, the risk for DIONJ begins with the fourth dose and increases with each dose beyond that. This early development of risk is because the IV route of a bisphosphonate loads the bone 140 times greater and faster than the oral route.[9] The similar risk profile for a once-per-year IV bisphosphonate dosing versus a once-per-month dosing is due to the 11.2-year half-life in bone (Fig 1-5a; see Table 1-2).

> The IV route of a bisphosphonate loads the bone 140 times greater and faster than the oral route.[9]

For denosumab, the subcutaneous route of administration is the same for osteopenia/osteoporosis patients as it is for cancer patients. Here the difference in toxicity is related to the dose (60 mg vs 120 mg) and the frequency of administration (once every 6 months vs once per month; see Table 1-2).

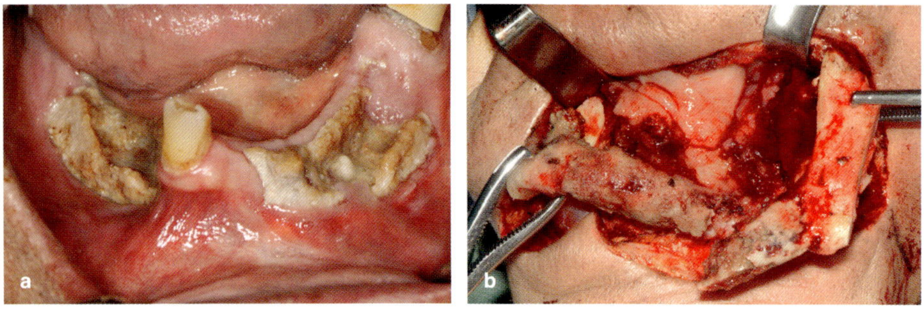

FIG 1-5 *(a)* Stage III DIONJ due to IV zoledronate at 5 mg/year after six doses. *(b)* Extensive Stage III DIONJ with a pathologic fracture due to denosumab administered as a replacement for zoledronate.

7. Heightened risk when denosumab follows a bisphosphonate

With the more recent marketing of denosumab and the known risks for DIONJ from bisphosphonates throughout the medical profession, many treating physicians have switched from a bisphosphonate to denosumab in both osteopenia/osteoporosis patients and cancer patients. However, the loading of alveolar bone with a bisphosphonate by either the oral or IV route followed by subcutaneous denosumab has resulted in a rapid development of a more extensive and more severe form of DIONJ with advanced staging (Fig 1-5b).

Initiating factors

Factors too often touted as risk factors are actually initiating factors. That is, these entities do not cause DIONJ by themselves, but the increased need for bone remodeling and renewal created by these factors can initiate DIONJ in a person taking or who has taken one of the known drugs that cause DIONJ.

Extractions

The greatest initiator of DIONJ is a tooth extraction (61%; Table 1-3).[9,25] In a person within the risk category for DIONJ, the extraction of a tooth creates an increased need for bone turnover, which the alveolar bone may not be able to meet depending on the level of risk within the alveolar bone as discussed in this section. In some cases, the extraction occurs within already necrotic bone that may not be overtly exposed. That is, in some cases the necrotic bone is only exposed by a subtle pinpoint fistula or through the furcation of a molar tooth or subtly via the periodontal ligament space before the tooth is extracted. Therefore, it may be best to say that an extraction is associated with

> The greatest initiator of DIONJ is a tooth extraction.

Table 1-3 Associated indicators of DIONJ (N = 400)

Indicator	N	Percentage of cases
Tooth removal	244	61%
Spontaneous/occlusion	112	28%
Dental implant placement	20	5%
Periodontal surgery	20	5%
Other	4	1%

the identification of and diagnosis of DIONJ in 61% of cases, where in some cases the trauma from the extraction initiated it while in other cases the DIONJ was already present.

Traumatic occlusion/spontaneous

In the author's experience, about 30% of DIONJ seems to occur without any extraction of teeth or surgical intrusion into the alveolar bone. Although necrotic bone in the jaws may develop directly related to the potency and the length of time of taking the drug, on closer inspection most are seen to be related to traumatic occlusion. It is noted that 50% of DIONJ cases from any drug occur in the posterior lingual area of the mandible, where the wide occlusal table of molars and the axial loading of occlusal forces is directed onto the lingual cortex (Figs 1-6a and 1-6b). In these same cases, the wear pattern and admitted bruxing habits of some patients is often seen as well (Fig 1-6c). Similarly, DIONJ is often targeted to areas of selective occlusion due to missing teeth or restorations in hyperocclusion (Figs 1-6d and 1-6e).

DIONJ is often targeted to areas of selective occlusion due to missing teeth or restorations in hyperocclusion.

Chronic inflammation

No doubt chronic inflammation from untreated periodontal disease is an initiating factor or contributes to another initiating factor (ie, traumatic occlusion or an extraction to create DIONJ). Inflammation increases the osteoclast-mediated turnover rate of alveolar bone that causes the bone to die off if it is loaded with a bisphosphonate or if the osteoclast population is diminished by denosumab.

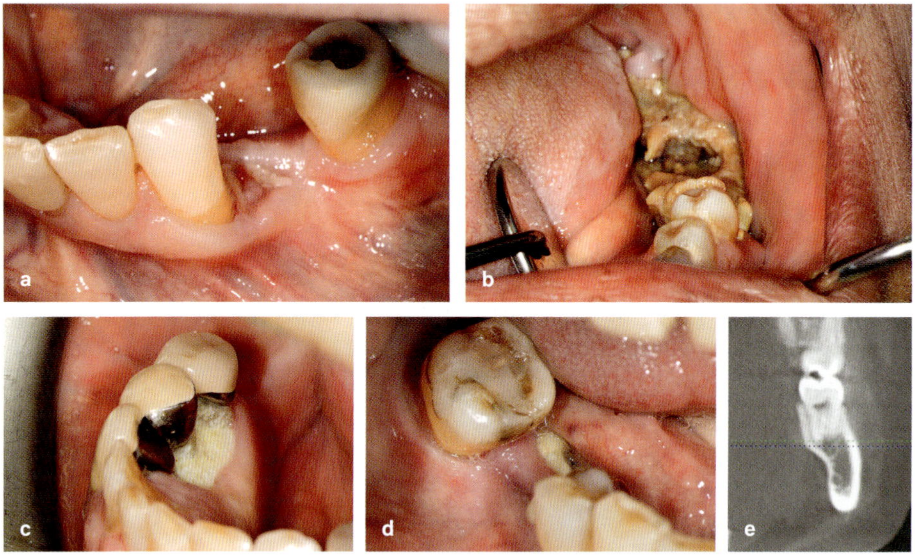

FIG 1-6 *(a)* DIONJ initiated after a periodontal osseous surgery. *(b)* DIONJ initiated by a tooth extraction. *(c)* Clinical DIONJ is most often seen on the lingual cortex opposite the molars. *(d)* DIONJ adjacent to the molar with obvious severe wear. *(e)* The axial loading of molars is directed on the lingual cortex and is responsible for the high incidence of DIONJ in that location.

Surgical intrusion into alveolar bone

Like tooth extractions, several dental procedures have been known to result in DIONJ (Fig 1-7a). Procedures such as alveolar bone biopsies (Fig 1-7b), crown lengthening (Fig 1-7c), osseous periodontal surgery, and the placement of dental implants (Fig 1-7d) have resulted in DIONJ by imparting a degree of trauma to the alveolar bone that in turn creates a need for bone remodeling and renewal, which these drugs inhibit.

Vulnerable sites

Areas of common occurrence of DIONJ have also been incorrectly labeled as risk factors. Once again, these areas do not develop necrotic bone by themselves. It is another underlying injury that causes these areas to become necrotic (ie, radiation, bisphosphonates, RANK ligand inhibitors, and more rarely antiangiogenic drugs). The most common vulnerable site is the posterior lingual cortex of the mandible (Fig 1-8a).

The most common vulnerable site is the posterior lingual cortex of the mandible.

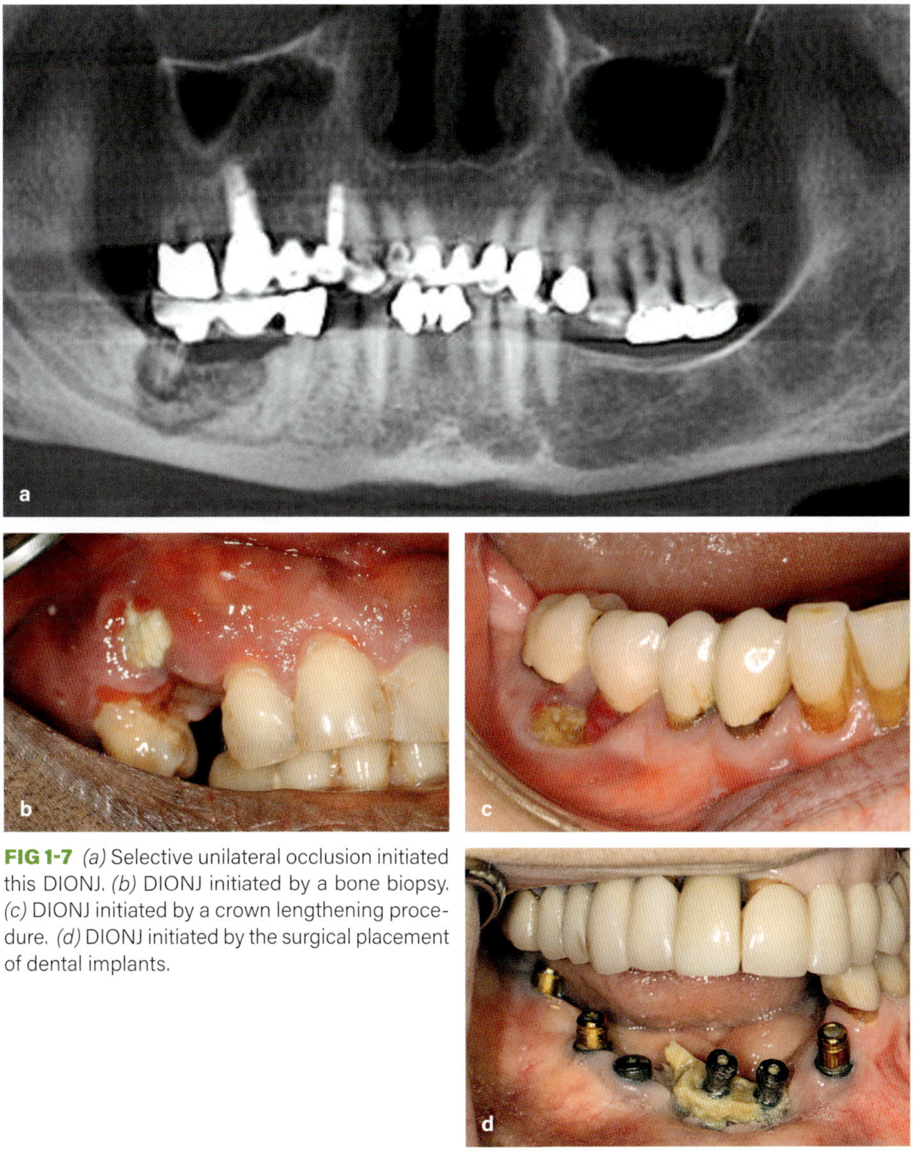

FIG 1-7 *(a)* Selective unilateral occlusion initiated this DIONJ. *(b)* DIONJ initiated by a bone biopsy. *(c)* DIONJ initiated by a crown lengthening procedure. *(d)* DIONJ initiated by the surgical placement of dental implants.

Another well-known vulnerable site is the surface of a torus (Fig 1-8b). Although we recognize that tori are hard mature outcroppings of compact bone, it is often unappreciated that they have a high turnover rate particularly at their surface. The vulnerability of tori to develop DIONJ is added to by the thin oral mucosa that overlays them. Additionally, in the author's experience, DIONJ develops in the mandible twice as frequently as in the maxilla.

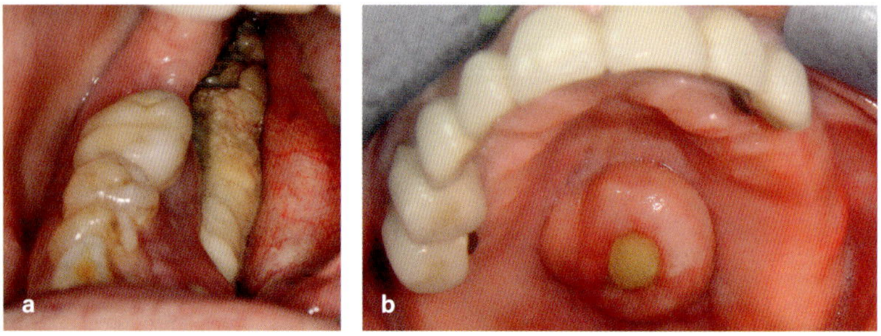

FIG 1-8 *(a)* The most common site for DIONJ is the posterior mandibular lingual cortex. *(b)* Tori are a frequent site for DIONJ.

Comorbidities

The many comorbidities often incorrectly labeled as risk factors also do not cause DIONJ by themselves. They certainly contribute to it by making DIONJ occur sooner or to become more extensive and severe when it does occur. Some of these comorbidities include diabetes, smoking, cancer, corticosteroids, chemotherapy, and immune-based diseases, among others.[12–14]

Definition of DIONJ

Despite its many names, the definition of DIONJ is mostly consistent among the position papers produced by various originations.[5,26,27] A good working definition is this:

> Exposed nonhealing bone in the mandible or maxilla that is present for more than 8 weeks in a person who received a systemic drug known to cause ONJ but who has not received a local tumoricidal dose of radiation to the jaws.

Staging of DIONJ

Staging systems for oral cancer,[28] lymphomas,[29] and osteoradionecrosis[30] identify the severity and extent of the disease and guide treatment decisions and prognosis. None of them include the subjective relation of pain, which is variable between patients and based on analgesic use. The following is a straightforward staging system for DIONJ developed by the author:

- **Stage 0:** Radiographic and/or clinical evidence of alveolar bone toxicity without bone exposure. This is often recognized as sclerosis of the lamina dura and widening of the periodontal ligament space. It is often noted symptomatically as

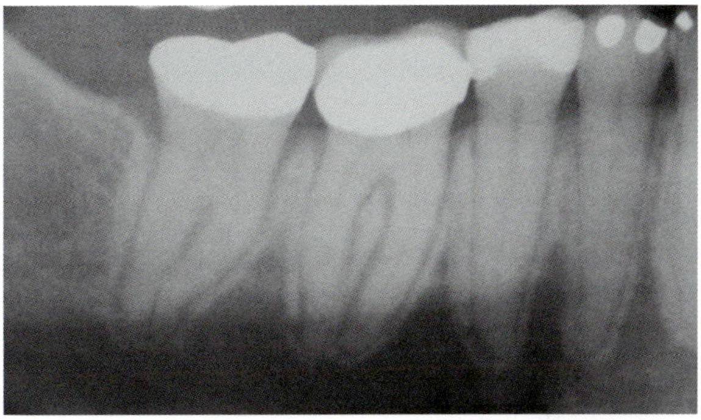

FIG 1-9 Sclerosis of the lamina dura and a widened periodontal ligament space.

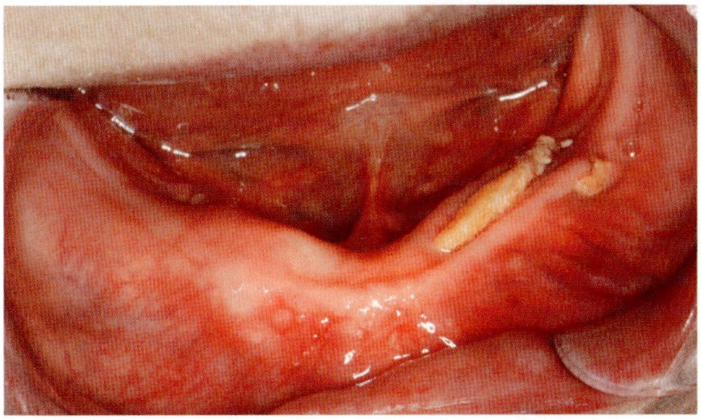

FIG 1-10 Stage I DIONJ.

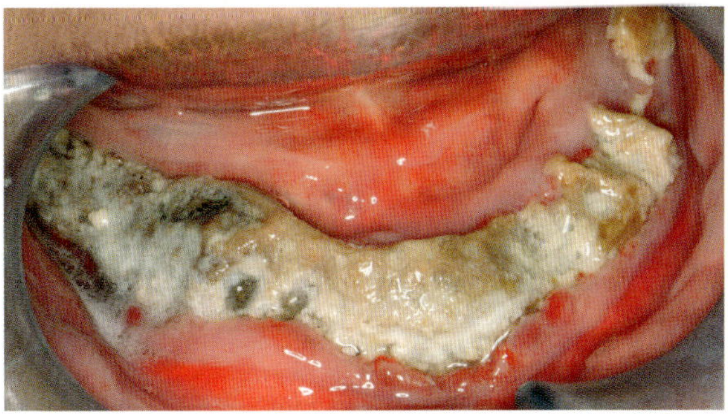

FIG 1-11 Stage II DIONJ.

deep bone pain or tooth pain or tooth mobility not attributed to a more obvious cause (Fig 1-9). Stage 0 should be taken as caution that exposed bone may result if subjected to any one of the initiating factors discussed.

- **Stage I:** Exposed bone limited to one quadrant (Fig 1-10)
- **Stage II:** Exposed bone in two quadrants (Fig 1-11)
- **Stage III:** Exposed bone in three or four quadrants (Figs 1-12a and 1-12b) **OR** osteolysis to the inferior border of the mandible (Fig 1-12c) **OR** pathologic fracture (Fig 1-12d) **OR** extension into the maxillary sinus (Fig 1-12e)

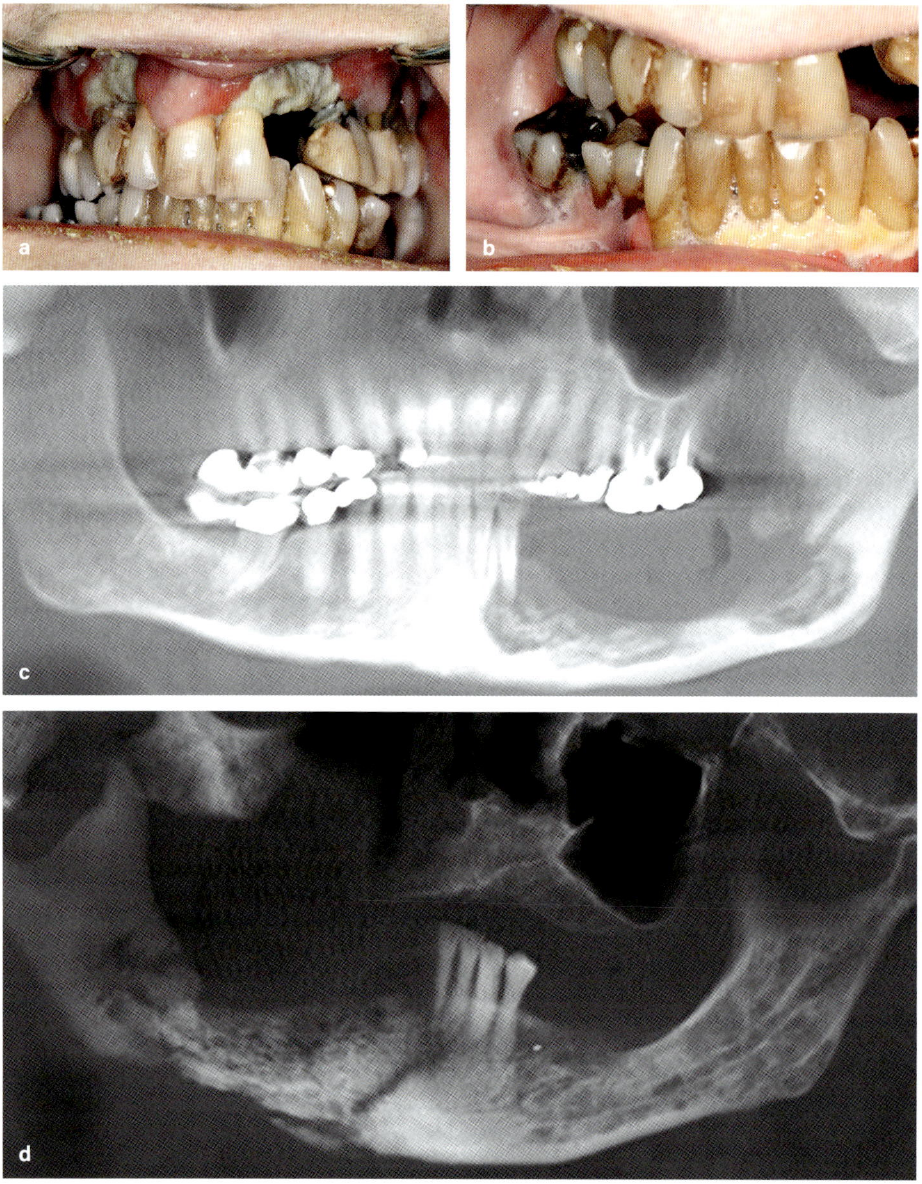

FIG 1-12 Stage III DIONJ. *(a and b)* Three separate areas of DIONJ. *(c)* Osteolysis to the inferior border. *(d)* Pathologic fracture.

Antiangiogenic Drugs

Pertinent only to patients being treated for cancer are two other drugs known to cause DIONJ: bevacizumab[31] and sunitinib.[32] Bevacizumab is used in the treatment of lung cancer and is a direct inhibitor of vascular endothelial growth factor (VEGF).[33] It is usually administered IV based upon weight but most commonly 500 mg every

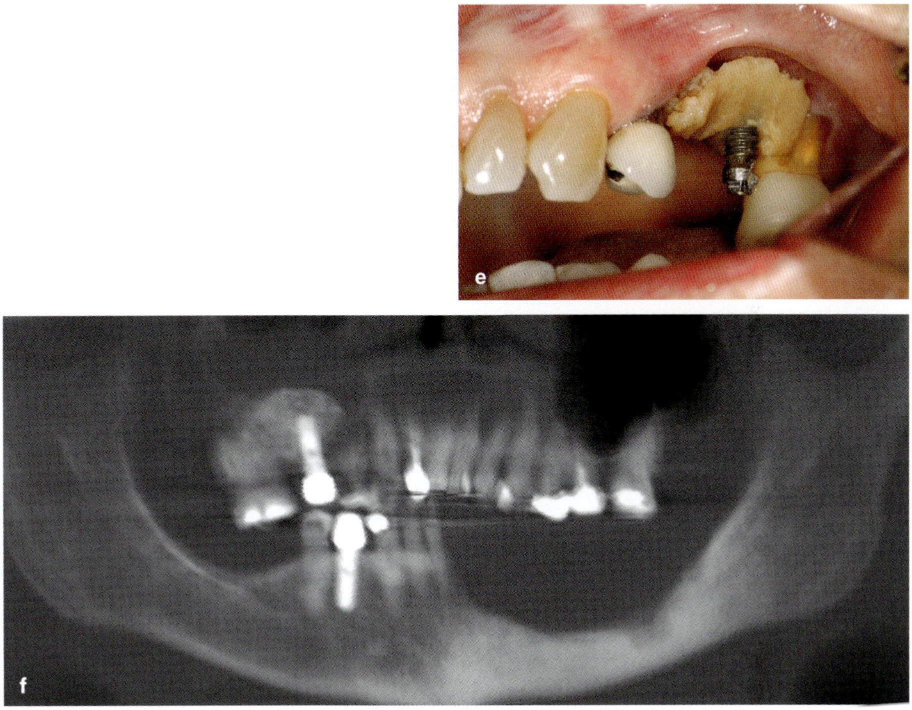

FIG 1-12 (*cont*) *(e and f)* Maxillary sinus involvement.

2 weeks. Reported cases of DIONJ from this drug and those observed by the author have mostly been Stage I and respond to discontinuation (drug holiday) with either stabilization, sequestration, or local surgical removal (Fig 1-13).

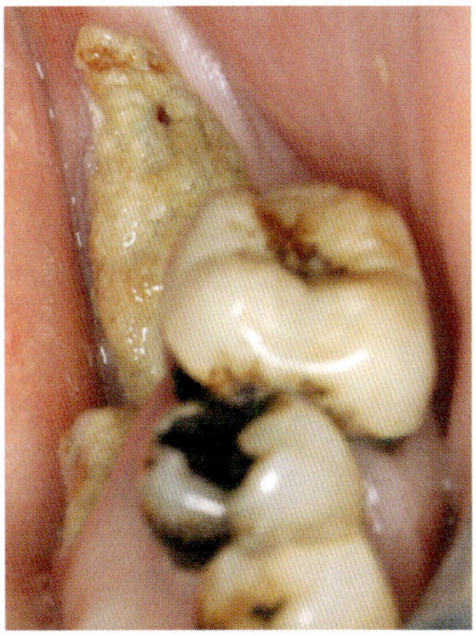

FIG 1-13 DIONJ caused by bevacizumab.

Sunitinib is a tyrosine kinase inhibitor mostly administered to patients with renal cancer and less commonly for gastrointestinal stroma tumors and pancreatic neuroendocrine tumors.[34] It inhibits several growth factors required by the cancer but seems to have its most profound effect on VEGF and therefore is mostly an antiangiogenic drug. Sunitinib has more reported cases of DIONJ than bevacizumab and produces more Stage II and Stage III presentations (Fig 1-14). It is an oral drug taken as a daily dose between 12.5 mg and 50 mg for nine 6-week cycles. Discontinuation of the drug seems to halt the progression of DIONJ, and most cases are either stabilized with exposed bone or require surgical removal including resections if extensive.

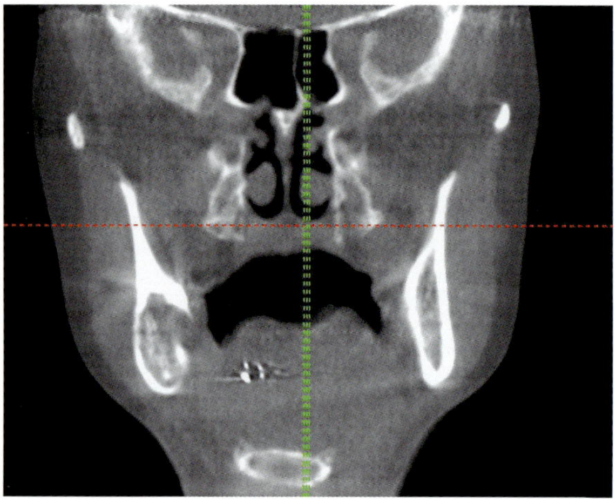

FIG 1-14 DIONJ caused by sunitinib.

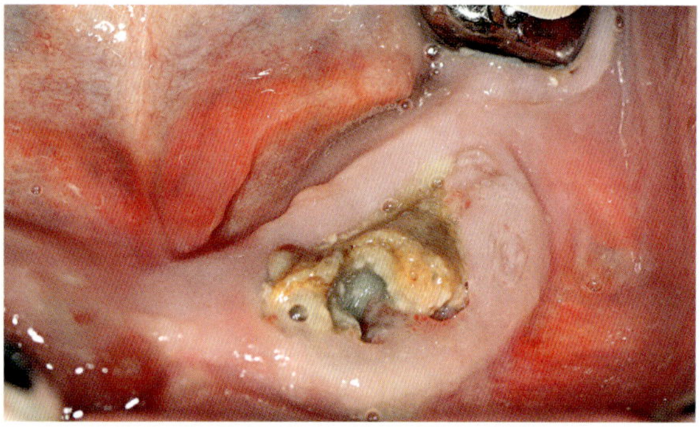

FIG 1-15 DIONJ resulting from tocilizumab prescribed to treat rheumatoid arthritis.

Drugs prescribed for immune-based disease

In rare instances, the drug tocilizumab has caused DIONJ cases (Fig 1-15). Tocilizumab is an interleukin-6 (IL-6) inhibitor used to treat rheumatoid arthritis, giant cell arteritis, and some juvenile polyarthritis conditions.[35,36] As an IL-6 inhibitor, it represents a specific inhibitor of immune-based inflammation but also an inhibitor of osteoclast development similar but not identical to denosumab as a RANK ligand inhibitor. The inhibition of IL-6 prevents the mononuclear precursors cells of osteoclasts from fusing together to produce a multinucleated cell and therefore stops the development of osteoclasts resulting in a risk for DIONJ.

Tocilizumab may be administered subcutaneously but is mostly infused IV at 4 mg/kg per week for 4 weeks followed by 8 mg/kg per week for another 4 weeks. Discontinuation of the drug halts the progression of DIONJ, but the few cases experienced by the author have been Stage III, requiring a resection.

References

1. World Health Organization. ICD-10: International Statistical Classification of Diseases and Related Health Problems, 10th Revision. https://icd.who.int/browse10/2019/en. Accessed 3 March 2021.
2. Marx RE. Pamidronate (Aredia) and zoledronate (Zometa) induced avascular necrosis of the jaws: A growing epidemic. J Oral Maxillofac Surg 2003;61:1115–1117.
3. Wang J, Goodger NM, Pogrel MA. Osteonecrosis of the jaws associated with cancer chemotherapy. J Oral Maxillofac Surg 2003;61:1104–1107.
4. Rosella D, Papi P, Giardino R, Cicalini E, Piccoli L, Pompa G. Medication-related osteonecrosis of the jaw: Clinical and practical guidelines. J Int Soc Prev Community Dent 2016;6:97–104.
5. Edwards BJ, Hellstein JW, Jacobsen PL, Kaltman S, Mariotti A, Migliorati CA. Updated recommendations for managing the care of patients receiving oral bisphosphonate therapy: An advisory statement from the American Dental Association Council on Scientific Affairs. American Dental Association Council on Scientific Affairs Expert Panel on Bisphosphonate-Associated Osteonecrosis of the Jaw. J Am Dent Assoc 2008;139:1674–1677.
6. Hellstein JW, Marek CL. Bisphosphonate osteochemonecrosis (bis-phossy jaw): Is this phossy jaw of the 21st century? J Oral Maxillofac Surg 2005;63:682–689.
7. Buckley KA, Fraser WD. Receptor activator for nuclear factor kappaB ligand and osteoprotegerin: Regulators of bone physiology and immune responses/potential therapeutic agents and biochemical markers. Ann Clin Biochem 2002;39(pt 6):551–556.
8. Dixon RB, Tricker ND, Geretto LP. Bone turnover in early canine mandible and tibia [abstract 2549]. J Dent Res 1997;76:336.
9. Marx RE. Oral and Intravenous Bisphosphonate-Induced Osteonecrosis of the Jaws: History, Etiology, Prevention, and Treatment, ed 2. Chicago: Quintessence, 2011:45–89.
10. Neviaser AS, Lane JM, Lenart BA, Edobor-Osula F, Lorich DG. Low-energy femoral shaft fractures associated with alendronate use. J Orthop Trauma 2008;22:346–350.
11. Black DM, Kelly MP, Genant HK, et al. Bisphosphonates and fractures of the subtrochanteric or diaphyseal femur. Fracture Intervention Trial Steering Committee; HORIZON Pivotal Fracture Trial Steering Committee. N Engl J Med 2010;362:1761–1771.
12. Wessel JH, Dodson TB, Zavras A. Zoledronate, smoking, and obesity are strong risk factors for osteonecrosis of the jaw: A case-control study. J Oral Maxillofac Surg 2008;66:625–631.
13. Ruggiero S, Gralow J, Marx RE, et al. Practical guidelines for the prevention, diagnosis, and treatment of osteonecrosis of the jaw in patients with cancer. J Oncol Pract 2006;2:7–14.
14. Rahimi-Nedjat RK, Sagheb K, Pabst A, Olk L, Walter C. Diabetes mellitus and its association to the occurrence of medication-related osteonecrosis of the jaw. Dent J (Basel) 2016;4:17.
15. Lasseter KC, Porras AG, Denker A, Santhanagopal A, Daifotis A. Pharmacokinetic considerations in determining the terminal elimination half-lives of bisphosphonates. Clin Drug Investig 2005;25:107–114.
16. Josse R, Khan A, Ngui D, Shapiro M. Denosumab, a new pharmacotherapy option for postmenopausal osteoporosis. Curr Med Res Opin 2013;29:1211.
17. Lacey DL, Boyle WJ, Simonet WS, et al. Bench to bedside: Elucidation of the OPG-RANK-RANKL pathway and the development of denosumab. Nat Rev Drug Discov 2012;11:401–419.
18. Russell RG, Croucher PI, Rogers MJ. Bisphosphonates: Pharmacology, mechanisms of action and clinical uses. Osteoporos Int 1999;9(suppl 2):S66–S80.
19. Cardwell CR, Abnet CC, Cantwell MM, Murray LJ. Exposure to oral bisphosphonates and risk of esophageal cancer. JAMA 2010;304:657–663.
20. Edwards BJ, Usmani S, Raisch DW, et al. Acute kidney injury and bisphosphonate use in cancer: A report from the research on adverse drug events and reports (RADAR) project. J Oncol Pract 2013;9:101–106.
21. Glowacki J. Bisphosphonates and bone. Ortho J Harvard Med School 2005;7:64–67.
22. Coxon FP, Thompson K, Roelofs AJ, Ebetino FH, Rogers MJ. Visualizing mineral binding and uptake of bisphosphonate by osteoclasts and non-resorbing cells. Bone 2008;42:848–860.
23. Bone HG, Bolognese MA, Yuen CK, et al. Effects of denosumab on bone mineral density and bone turnover in postmenopausal women. J Clin Endocrinol Metab 2008;93:2149–2157.
24. Boyce BF, Xing L. Biology of RANK, RANKL, and osteoprotegerin. Arthritis Res Ther 2007;9(suppl 1):S1.

25. Marx RE, Sawatari Y, Fortin M, Broumand V. Bisphosphonate-induced exposed bone (osteonecrosis/osteopetrosis) of the jaws: Risk factors, recognition, prevention, and treatment. J Oral Maxillofac Surg 2005;63:1567–1575.
26. Advisory Task Force on Bisphosphonate-Related Osteonecrosis of the Jaws, American Association of Oral and Maxillofacial Surgeons. American Association of Oral and Maxillofacial Surgeons position paper on bisphosphonate-related osteonecrosis of the jaws. J Oral Maxillofac Surg 2007;65:369–376.
27. Khosla S, Burr D, Cauley J, et al; American Society for Bone and Mineral Research. Bisphosphonate-associated osteonecrosis of the jaw: Report of a task force of the American Society for Bone and Mineral Research. J Bone Miner Res 2007;22:1479–1491.
28. American Cancer Society. Oral Cavity (Mouth) and Oropharyngeal (Throat) Cancer. https://www.cancer.org/cancer/oral-cavity-and-oropharyngeal-cancer.html. Accessed 3 March 2021.
29. American Cancer Society. Non-Hodgkin Lymphoma (Adults). https://www.cancer.org/cancer/non-hodgkin-lymphoma.html. Accessed 3 March 2021.
30. Marx RE, Stern DS. Oral and Maxillofacial Pathology: A Rationale for Diagnosis and Treatment, ed 2. Chicago: Quintessence, 2012.
31. Guarneri V, Miles D, Robert N, et al. Bevacizumab and osteonecrosis of the jaw: Incidence and association with bisphosphonate therapy in three large prospective trials in advanced breast cancer. Breast Cancer Res Treat 2010;122:181–188.
32. Fleissig Y, Regev E, Lehman H. Sunitinib related osteonecrosis of jaw: A case report. Oral Surg Oral Med Oral Pathol Oral Radiol 2012;113:e1–e3.
33. dos Santos LV, Cruz MR, de Lima Lopes G, da Silveira Nogueira Lima JP. VEGF-A levels in bevacizumab-treated breast cancer patients: A systematic review and meta-analysis. Breast Cancer Res Treat 2015;151:481–489.
34. Tourneau CL, Raymond E, Faivre S. Sunitinib: A novel tyrosine kinase inhibitor. A brief review of its therapeutic potential in the treatment of renal carcinoma and gastrointestinal stromal tumors (GIST). Ther Clin Risk Manag 2007;3:341–348.
35. Genovese MC, McKay JD, Nasonov EL, et al. Interleukin-6 receptor inhibition with tocilizumab reduces disease activity in rheumatoid arthritis with inadequate response to disease-modifying antirheumatic drugs: The tocilizumab in combination with traditional disease-modifying antirheumatic drug therapy study. Arthritis Rheum 2008;58:2968–2980.
36. De Benedetti F, Brunner HI, Ruperto N, et al; PRINTO; PRCSG. Randomized trial of tocilizumab in systemic juvenile idiopathic arthritis. N Engl J Med 2012;367:2385–2395.

Chapter 2

Prevention and Management of DIONJ in Patients Treated for Osteopenia/ Osteoporosis

What Is Osteoporosis?

Osteoporosis is a disease whereby bone loses some of its cortical thickness and the medullary trabecular struts between the cortices become thin and disconnected (Fig 2-1). Therefore, the bone becomes porotic and weaker and may fracture, leading to complications from these fractures. Osteoporosis affects every bone in the skeleton, but the bones most susceptible to fracture and thereby where fracture prevention via medication is most focused are the vertebral bodies (often incorrectly termed "spinal fractures"), the head of the femur (often incorrectly termed "hip fractures"), and the wrist area (the distal radius or ulna).

Osteoporosis is diagnosed via a radiologic system called a DEXA scan (dual-energy x-ray absorptiometry) that gives a bone mineral density (BMD) number in g/cm^2. This value is similar to the Hounsfield density evaluations many dentists make on their CBCT scans. The BMD is converted to a T-score, which is used to arrive at a diagnosis of either normal bone density, osteopenia, or actual osteoporosis. The T-score is a comparison of the bone density in the tested patient to the World Health Organization's database for the average bone density of a 22-year-old white woman. Therefore, nearly every T-score will be presented as a negative number, which represents the number of standard deviations of the patient's BMD from the average value of a 22-year-old white woman. A T-score greater than –1 is considered normal; T-scores between –1 and –2.5 diagnose osteopenia; and a T-score less than –2.5 diagnoses osteoporosis. Severe osteoporosis is the diagnosis given if the T-score is less than –2.5 and the patient exhibits a "fragility fracture" (Fig 2-2). It is useful for dental practitioners to be familiar with these diagnostic criteria and stratification of osteoporosis so as to be conversant with the physician's prescribing osteopenia/osteoporosis drugs, some of which cause DIONJ.

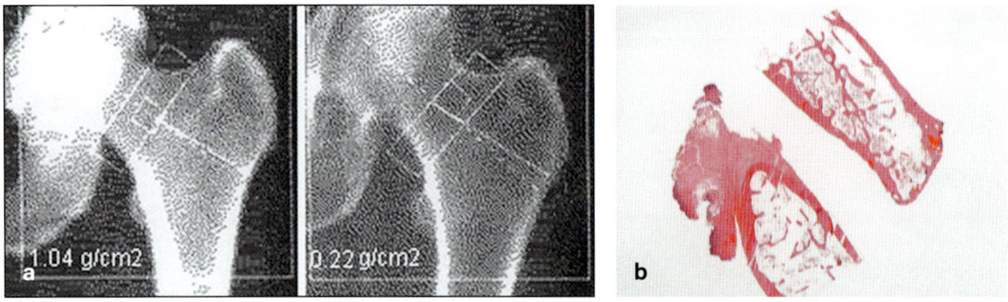

FIG 2-1 *(a)* Radiograph of a hip joint in a patient without osteoporosis *(left)* compared to a radiograph of a hip joint in a patient with osteoporosis *(right)*. Note the greater degree of bone mineral density in the latter. (Courtesy of Susan Ott, MD, University of Washington.) *(b)* Histologic sections of a vertebra and a mandible from an osteoporotic woman showing thinner cortices and trabecular bone as well as breaks and disconnects of the cortical struts (hematoxylin-eosin [h&e] staining).

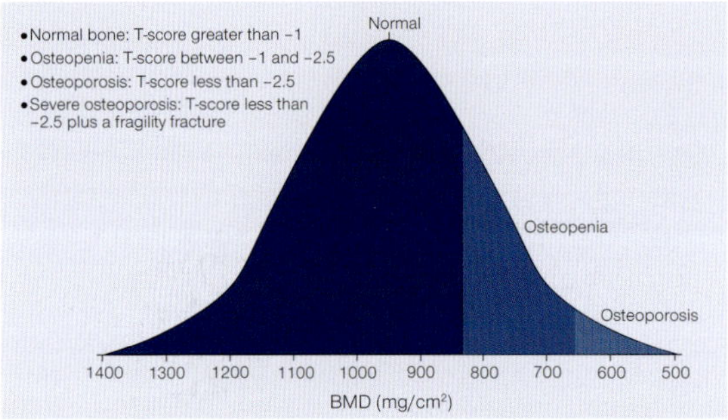

FIG 2-2 The World Health Organization defines osteopenia and osteoporosis based on BMD values. *Osteopenia* is defined as a BMD that is between 1 and 2.5 standard deviations from the maximum mean bone density for a 22-year-old white woman (ie, T-score of −1 to −2.5), and *osteoporosis* is defined as a BMD that is more than 2.5 standard deviations from the maximum mean bone density (ie, T-score less than −2.5). (Courtesy of Susan Ott, MD, University of Washington.)

> Osteopenia and osteoporosis are most common in post-menopausal women.

Who Develops Osteopenia/Osteoporosis?

Osteopenia and osteoporosis are most common in postmenopausal women, men and women taking long-term corticosteroids, and women with non-metastatic breast cancer taking steroid medications that induce osteopenia/osteoporosis or certain chemotherapy drugs termed *aromatase inhibitors*.

Postmenopausal osteoporosis

The systemic decline in estrogen production after menopause begins a slow progression of osteopenia to osteoporosis in many women. This is largely due to the fact that estrogen is required for osteoblast differentiation. Osteopenia and osteoporosis result by the natural cycle of bone turnover, where new bone formation cannot keep up with the osteoclast-mediated bone resorption. That is, as 100 g of bone is naturally resorbed as part of the normal bone turnover cycle, only 96 to 98 g is resynthesized. As years progress, this slight but continuous bone loss becomes significant, resulting in porotic bone with reduced fracture resistance.

The often-promoted theory that osteoclasts are overly active after menopause is incorrect, as few if any normal cellular functions increase with age—ie, men do not get more hair as they age and the pigment cells of hair follicles do not overact to make our hair darker. Instead, less hair redevelops to replace that which is lost, and the remaining hair turns gray. Similarly, muscle mass and neurologic functions do not improve beyond 40 years of age.

Postmenopausal osteoporosis remains an imbalance between a normal bone resorption rate and a reduced bone resynthesis rate. Within this group, white women and Asian women seem to have a greater genetic predilection for osteopenia/osteoporosis, while black women and men of any race have less.

Postmenopausal osteoporosis remains an imbalance between a normal bone resorption rate and a reduced bone resynthesis rate.

Steroid-induced osteopenia/osteoporosis

Steroid-induced osteopenia/osteoporosis reminds us that bone is more than a mineralized tissue and that the BMD and T-score studies do not actually describe the full picture of bone strength. Bone is mostly type 1 collagen that is in a tightly bound triple helix with hydroxyapatite crystals embedded into it. Corticosteroids break down collagen for energy and therefore reduce total body collagen. This reduction in collagen and its breakdown in bone, followed by its removal from bone, results in less overall bone and a more mineralized and brittle bone with an increased fracture risk.

Aromatase inhibitor–induced osteopenia/osteoporosis

Breast cancer patients are frequently on chemotherapy protocols that include aromatase inhibitors such as anastrazole and letrozole, whether they have metastasis or not.[1–3] Aromatase inhibitors block the production of estrogen and will tend toward osteopenia/osteoporosis similar to that of a postmenopausal woman or will further the estrogen deficiency of a postmenopausal woman.[3]

Evaluating a Patient Being Treated for Osteopenia/ Osteoporosis

Although no drug is approved by the US Food and Drug Administration (FDA) to treat osteopenia, many physicians prescribe DIONJ-causing drugs for this condition with the rationale of preventing osteoporosis. Based on the pharmacology and risks discussed in chapter 1, the following is the author's recommendation for a medical history questionnaire and review for such patients.

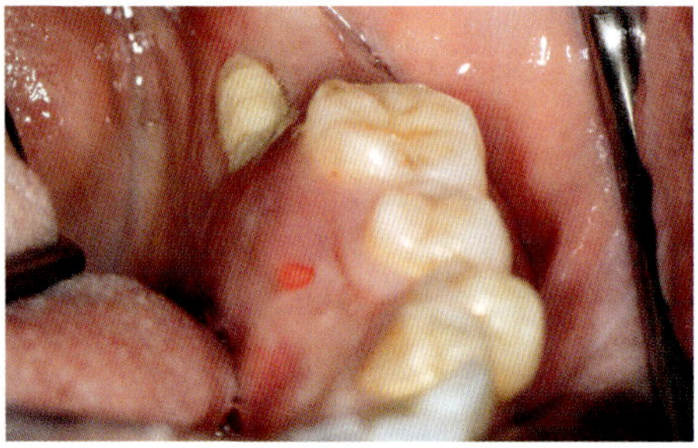

FIG 2-3 Many exposures of bone due to DIONJ can be noted by retracting the tongue to view the posterior mandibular cortex.

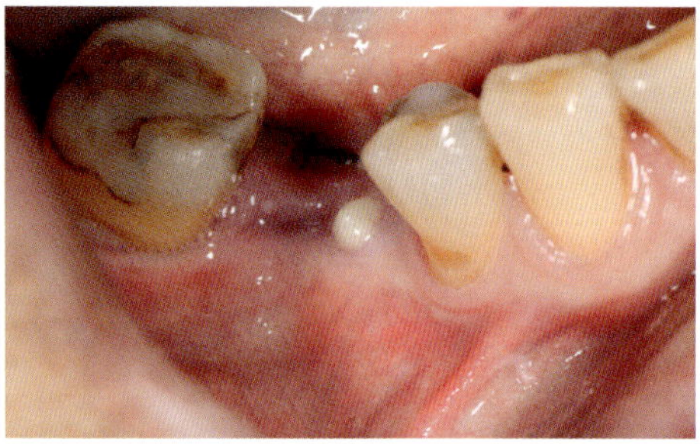

FIG 2-4 A subtle fistula identifies exposed bone, often with a larger amount of necrotic bone beneath the mucosa.

Suggested inclusions in your medical/dental history questionnaire

- Are you currently being treated for osteopenia or osteoporosis?
- Have you been treated for osteopenia or osteoporosis in the past?
- If so, do you recall the name of the medication? Was it a pill (alendronate, risedronate, or ibandronate)? Was it an injection under your skin (denosumab)? Was it an intravenous (IV) infusion once per year (zoledronate)?
- How long have you been taking the medication?
- When was the last time you took the medication or the medication was given to you?
- Do you have a known habit of tooth grinding?
- Do your teeth meet evenly?

Key examining points for patients being treated for osteopenia/osteoporosis

The key points in an oral clinical examination to assess for DIONJ are the following:

- Examine the posterior lingual areas thoroughly by retracting the tongue (Fig 2-3).
- Look for subtle or obvious areas of swelling, redness, granulation tissue, and fistulas under which exposed bone may exist (Fig 2-4).
- Examine each torus thoroughly if tori are present (Fig 2-5).
- Look for cutaneous fistulas (Fig 2-6).
- Examine for tooth mobility (Fig 2-7).
- Look for exposed bone in areas of recent oral surgery, especially extraction sockets (Fig 2-8).
- Carefully examine the occlusion, looking for excessive wear, premature contacts, and poorly fitting appliances (Fig 2-9).

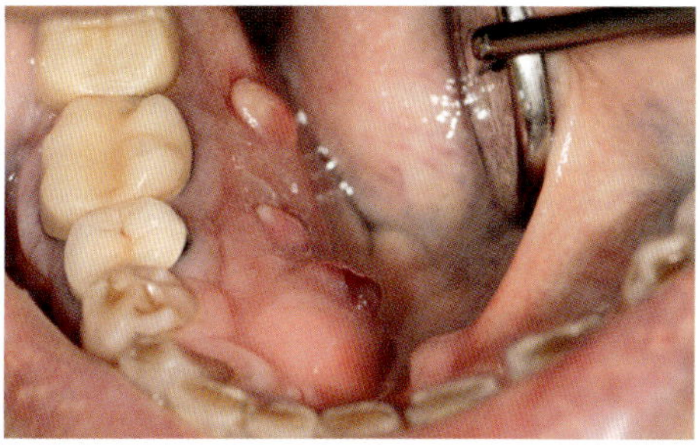

FIG 2-5 DIONJ on a torus.

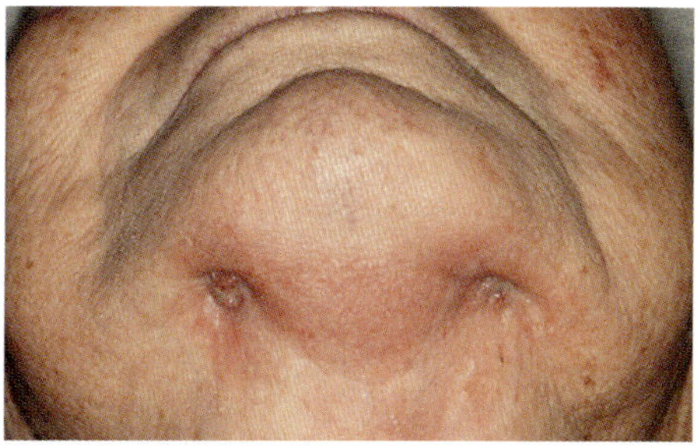

FIG 2-6 Cutaneous fistulas from DIONJ.

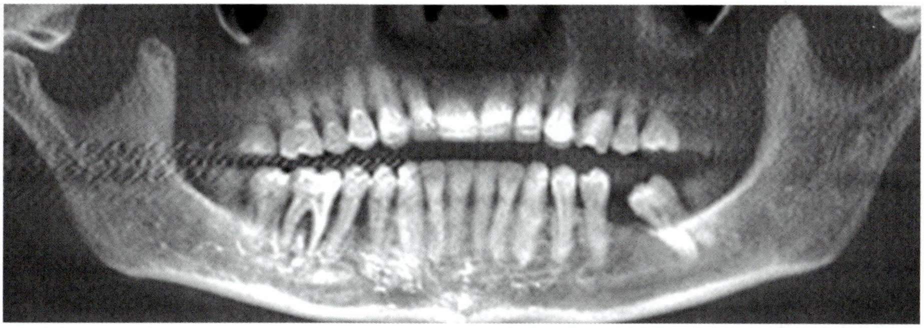

FIG 2-7 Tooth mobility due to bone loss from DIONJ.

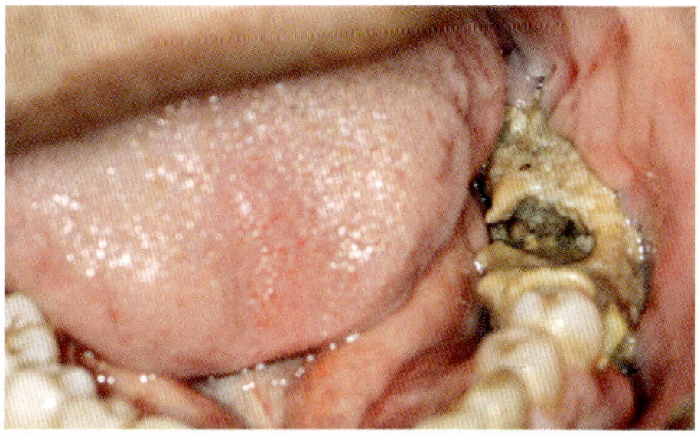

FIG 2-8 DIONJ identified by long-term nonhealing extraction sockets.

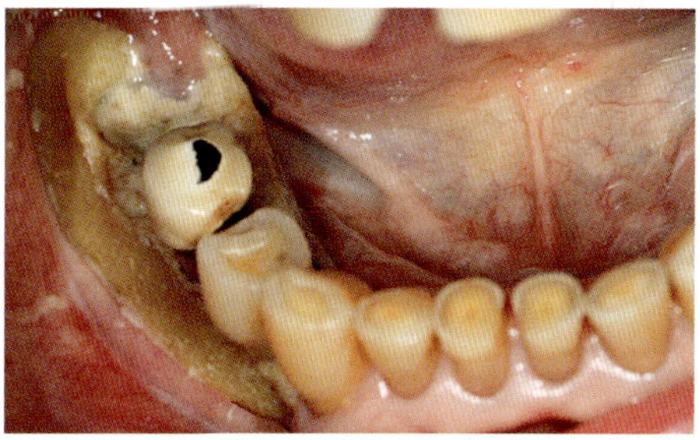

FIG 2-9 Be suspicious of developing or overt DIONJ if excessive tooth wear is noted during the examination.

Radiographic fine points to look for

Oral radiographs to assess for subtle or more obvious toxic effects of DIONJ-causing drugs is best accomplished with a CBCT scan. However, a technically well-performed plain panoramic film can be adequate as well. In any case, clinicians should look for the following:

- Sclerosis of the lamina dura (Fig 2-10)
- Diffuse areas of osteosclerosis (Fig 2-11)

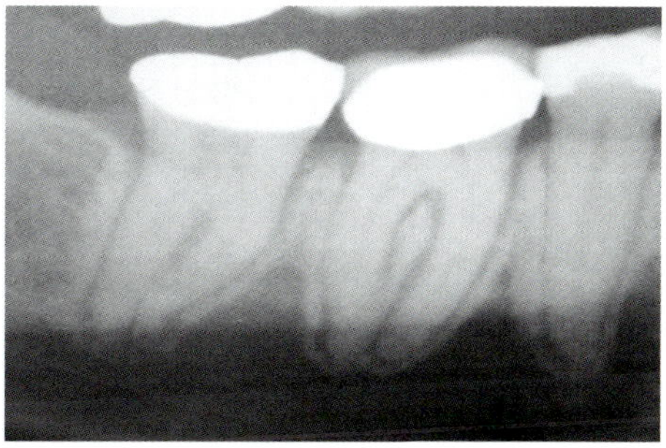

FIG 2-10 Sclerosis of the lamina dura in a patient who is currently taking or who has taken a drug known to cause DIONJ is a sign of Stage 0 DIONJ and should be viewed as a caution sign.

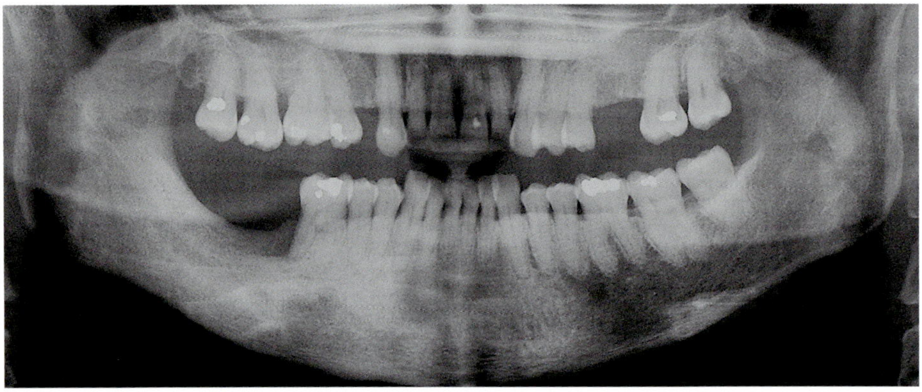

FIG 2-11 Diffuse areas of osteosclerosis seen in a patient who is currently taking or who has taken a drug known to cause DIONJ is indicative of the drug's negative effect on bone remodeling and renewal.

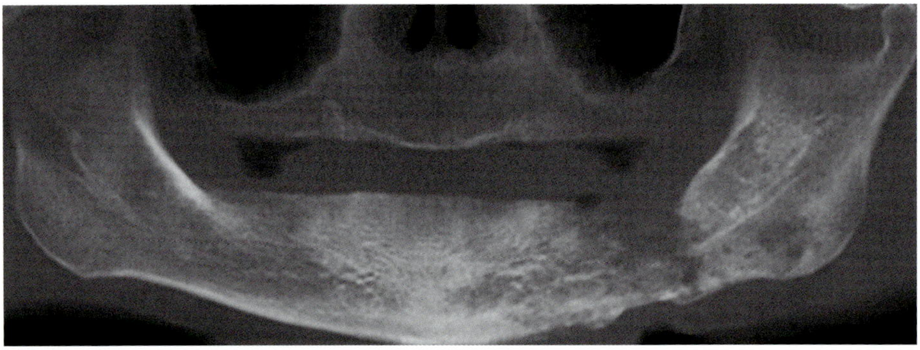

FIG 2-12 Osteolysis in DIONJ is a sign of bone mineral breakdown and also implies secondary infection.

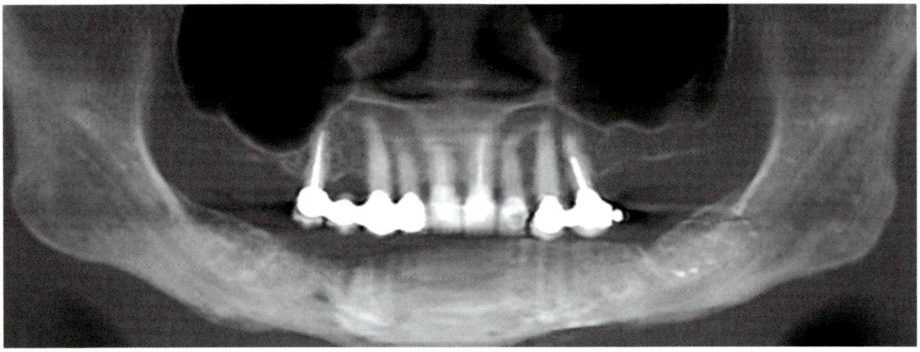

FIG 2-13 DIONJ-causing drugs negatively affect the bone remodel/renewal cycle mostly of the trabecular bone between the cortices. This can be seen as an area appearing differently from other trabecular bone areas.

- Areas of osteolysis (Fig 2-12)
- A disruption in the normal trabecular bone pattern (Fig 2-13)
- Irregularity or a beginning involucrum separating the lingual cortex in one or more areas of the mandible (Fig 2-14)

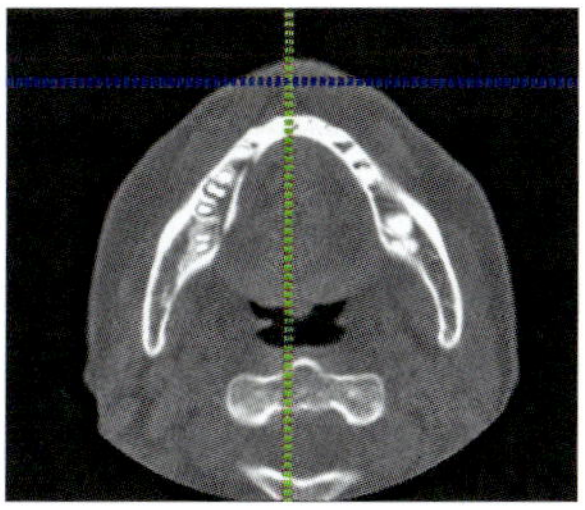

FIG 2-14 The lingual cortex is a target for DIONJ-causing drugs. The clinician is wise to look for signs of an involucrum separating the lingual cortex from the mandible.

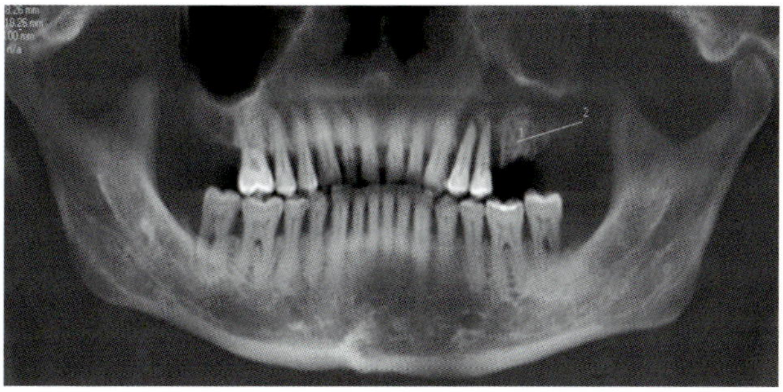

FIG 2-15 Irregularity of the maxillary sinus floor and/or an opacification of the sinus airspace in a patient who is currently taking or who has taken a drug known to cause DIONJ is suggestive of Stage III DIONJ.

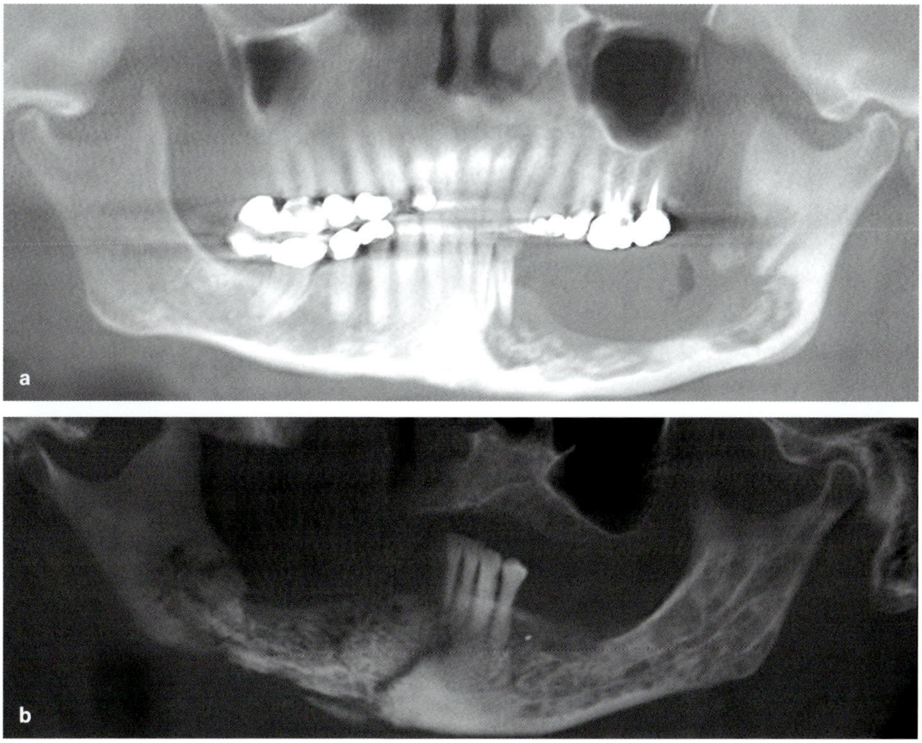

FIG 2-16 *(a)* Advanced Stage III DIONJ as seen by observing osteolysis to the inferior border of the mandible. *(b)* Advanced Stage III DIONJ as seen by observing a pathologic fracture of the mandible.

- A disruption in the floor of the maxillary sinus and/or an opacity within the maxillary sinus (Fig 2-15)
- Osteolysis extending to the inferior border of the mandible or a pathologic fracture (Fig 2-16)

Principles of Management

Patients with No Signs of DIONJ

- **Procedures noninvasive into bone are safe at all times:** ie, restorations, crowns, bridgework, partial dentures, complete dentures, dental prophylaxis, nonosseous periodontal procedures, coronal access root canal therapy.
- **Procedures at risk for DIONJ:** extractions, osseous periodontal surgery, bone biopsies, crown lengthening and dental implant surgery. Note that apicoectomies that approach the root apex from an alveolar bone–exposing flap are at risk for DIONJ. However, apicoectomies that approach the root apex from a vestibular approach are not at risk for DIONJ. Similarly Le Fort I osteotomies for orthognathic surgery are placed above the alveolar bone and are not at risk for DIONJ. Mandibular sagittal split osteotomies can be at risk if the more traditional Dal Pont modification is used due to the osteotomy involving the alveolar bone adjacent to the second molar. In such cases, the older and original osteotomy design that remains in the ramus and angle area of the mandible would be less of a risk for DIONJ.

Procedures noninvasive into bone are safe at all times.

- **Adult orthodontics:** During active treatment of osteopenia/osteoporosis with drugs that kill or inhibit osteoclasts (ie, bisphosphonates, denosumab, tocilizumab), the teeth will not move in response to orthodontic or Invisalign forces. In such cases, movement can be expected after a sufficient drug holiday has been observed.

A drug holiday is the most effective tool used to allow the continuation of dental/oral and maxillofacial surgical care with reduced risk for DIONJ in osteopenia/osteoporosis patients receiving one of the drugs known to cause DIONJ.

The basis and effective use of drug holidays

A drug holiday is the most effective tool used to allow the continuation of dental/oral and maxillofacial surgical care with reduced risk for DIONJ in osteopenia/osteoporosis patients receiving one of the drugs known to cause DIONJ. The length of the drug holiday required is specific for each drug and has been validated by the serum morning fasting C-terminal telopeptide test (CTX test)[4–6] and the experience of the author.

Oral bisphosphonate

The recommended drug holiday for a patient taking an oral bisphosphonate and who requires an invasive procedure into alveolar bone

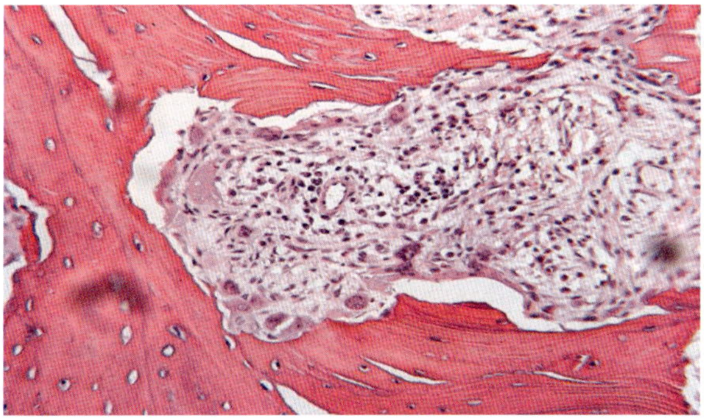

FIG 2-17 Actively resorbing osteoclasts with normal cytology are seen in a bone core biopsy after resolving DIONJ with a drug holiday.

as discussed in chapter 1 is 9 months prior to the procedure and 3 months after the procedure. The basis for this drug holiday is that despite the 11.2-year half-life of the oral bisphosphonates, the bone marrow stem cells and osteoclast precursors are able to repopulate a sufficient number of osteoclasts to remodel and renew bone as part of the healing process. This has been documented by a rise in the CTX values above 150 pg/dL after a drug holiday in all cases where the CTX test is not corrupted by either cancer, steroids, or methotrexate use.[3] It has also been verified by bone histology documenting the return of viable active osteoclasts after a drug holiday (Fig 2-17). This remarkable resilience of bone marrow has also been observed in bone marrow transplants after myeloablation for leukemia and multiple myeloma as well.[7]

In the patient who has taken an oral bisphosphonate, the drug holiday is effective by the fact that its low gut absorption allows the bone marrow to keep pace with the loss of osteoclasts directly from the drug. Essentially, the oral bisphosphonate has a trickle effect into the bone marrow that is 140 times less than the more overwhelming effect of an IV bisphosphonate, thus allowing the bone marrow to rebound and repopulate the lost osteoclasts from precursors. It also underscores the fact that drug holidays in cancer patients who have received IV zoledronate or IV pamidronate are ineffective due to their more rapid and greater loading of the bone and gradual depletion of bone marrow osteoclast precursors.

Denosumab

The recommended drug holiday for a patient taking subcutaneous denosumab 60 mg every 6 months for osteopenia/osteoporosis is quite different. It is 4 months prior and 3 months after a procedure invasive into alveolar bone. This somewhat shortened drug holiday balances the fact that denosumab is more toxic to the bone marrow osteoclast precursors but has a short half-life of just 26 days because it does not bind to bone as do bisphosphonates. This drug holiday only modifies the usual denosumab protocol for osteopenia/osteoporosis by 1 month.

Zoledronate

The recommended drug holiday for the less frequently used IV zoledronate protocol of 5 mg/year remains 9 months prior to the alveolar bone invasive procedure and 3 months afterward. Essentially, this regimen coincides well with the recommended drug administration schedule. That is, the planned procedure can be accomplished 9 months after the scheduled IV zoledronate infusion, and the 3-month postprocedure healing period is completed prior to the next scheduled dose.

How safe are drug holidays for the osteopenia/osteoporosis patient?

Drug holidays as described here are very safe and effective as documented by studies and the author's experience over the past 15 years. The sentinel study was a double-blind, prospective, placebo-controlled multicenter study.[8] In this study, 2,000 women were treated with alendronate for osteoporosis for 5 years. After the initial 5 years, half of the women were randomized to a placebo, while the other 1,000 women continued alendronate for another 5 years. The conclusions of this paper authored by twelve contributing centers are worth quoting:

> "Women who discontinued alendronate after 5 years showed a moderate decline in BMD and a gradual rise in biochemical markers [they used the serum CTX test] but no higher fracture risk other than for clinical vertebral fractures compared with those who continued alendronate. These results suggest that for many women, discontinuation of alendronate for up to 5 years does not appear to significantly increase fracture risk. However, women at very high risk of clinical cerebral fractures may benefit by continuing beyond 5 years."[8]

The drug holidays required by the dental profession are only 1 year at the most, compared to this study's discontinuation of alendronate for 5 years. Therefore, the drug holidays to be used as recommended in this text are a balance of maximum DIONJ risk aversion versus maintaining the benefits of the patient's osteopenia/osteoporosis treatment.

NOTE! The treatment of osteopenia/osteoporosis is not within the scope of the dental profession. All drug holidays should be instituted and administered by the prescribing physician. In the author's experience, physician colleagues are quite accepting and willing to work with a dental team and do not resist the utilization of a drug holiday. If, for some reason, a physician does not feel a drug holiday as suggested here is appropriate for their patient, they should be referred to the publication just quoted and offered the following list of alternative drugs used to treat osteopenia/osteoporosis with this DIONJ risk designation:

- **High risk:** Alendronate, 70 mg/wk po **OR** denosumab 60 mg/6 mo sc
- **Medium risk:** Zoledronate IV 5 mg/yr
- **Minimal risk:** Risedronate 35 mg/wk po **OR** ibandronate 150 mg/mo po
- **No risk:** Vitamin D3 and calcium **OR** raloxifene 60 mg/day po **OR** teriparatide (rhPTH 1-34) 20 mcg sc/day (limit to 2 years or less) **OR** abaloparatide (rhPTHI-80) 80 mcg sc/day (limit to 2 years or less) **OR** strontium renelate 2 g/day **OR** strontium citrate 680 mg/day

Patients with Exposed Bone (DIONJ) from an Osteopenia/ Osteoporosis Drug

In addition to the questions presented earlier in the chapter, the following questions should be asked during the medical history in the patient with clinical exposed bone:

- How long have you had the exposed bone?
- Are you still taking the medication we suspect is the cause?
- If you already stopped taking the osteopenia/osteoporosis medication, when was the last time you took it?
- Have you had a flare-up of increased pain and/or swelling?
- Do you have pain now?
- Have any medications like antibiotics been prescribed for your exposed bone? If it has, has it helped? Do you know the name of the medication?
- Have any debridement procedures been accomplished for you?
- Has any bone fallen out?
- Have you had radiation treatment for mouth cancer?

Nonsurgical management of DIONJ in the osteopenia/ osteoporosis patient

What to tell the patient

It is recommended to explain to the patient that the exposed bone is a direct complication of the osteopenia/osteoporosis drug and not any other drug or condition. It is also reasonable to explain that the drug has worked to prevent serious fractures of the spinal bones, hip, and wrist but that the jaws are 10 times

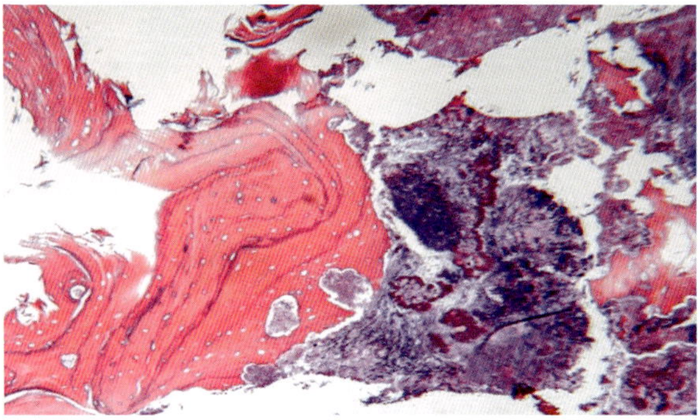

FIG 2-18 *Actinomyces* colonies on and within the crevices of necrotic bone from DIONJ.

more sensitive to these drugs, which is why the exposed bone only occurs in the jaws. Additionally, the author relates that because the exposed bone is "dead," it is not painful in and of itself; however, the exposed bone can become painful when the normal bacteria in the mouth colonize the bone or develop an infection in the bone. It is therefore important to control infection because infection will not only cause the patient pain but will also extend the area and amount of necrotic bone present. This straightforward explanation is greatly appreciated by the patient and improves their compliance with treatment.

The exposed bone can become painful when the normal bacteria in the mouth colonize the bone or develop an infection in the bone.

We further explain to the patient that treatment will require a drug holiday appropriate for the offending drug from their prescribing physician. We then begin them on an antibiotic regimen to control secondary infection during the drug holiday. The antibiotics used in this regimen can be taken long-term without significant side effects. If we prescribe an antibiotic known to have significant side effects if used long-term, we will limit it to 10 days. During the drug holiday, we look for a response and may then either continue long-term palliative care or recommend a bone removal procedure known as a *sequestrectomy* or less commonly a partial resection of the mandible or a sinus debridement if in the maxilla.

What antibiotic to use

Most every study has identified *Actinomyces* species to be the most common bacteria to colonize or infect exposed necrotic bone from DIONJ[9] (Fig 2-18). We have also found that *Moraxella*, *Eikenella*, and *Veillonella* species are often cocontaminants and/or infective agents together with *Actinomyces*. Therefore, penicillin derivatives are one of the two best choices of antibiotics that will provide the most predictable control of the infection and pain. The other antibiotic that has a good spectrum against these organisms is doxycycline. The added value of these two antibiotics is that they may be taken long-term without a high risk of toxicity or superinfection. Therefore, penicillin and doxycycline remain as the two frontline antibiotics to use. Although zithromycin and levofloxacin have proven effective in DIONJ cases as well, they are not useful on a long-term basis, zithromycin due to liver enzyme elevations and levofloxacin due to tendon weakness and rupture. Similarly, clindamycin has not proven to be effective due to the resistance of *Eikenella* species and the minimal sensitivity of *Actinomyces* to it.

Penicillin and doxycycline remain as the two frontline antibiotics to use.

The most effective initial antibiotic regimen in the face of exposed bone with drainage and pain is either amoxicillin 500 mg three times daily or doxycycline 100 mg once daily, with either combined with metronidazole 500 mg three times daily. The combination of either amoxicillin or doxycycline with metronidazole is most effective due to the sensitivity of the *Actinomyces* to amoxicillin and doxycycline and the sensitivity of the *Moraxella*, *Eikenella*, and *Veillonella* group to metronidazole. However, the author limits metronidazole to 14 days or fewer due to gastritis and abdominal discomfort if taken long-term. Following this initial double antibiotic treatment, amoxicillin or doxycycline can be continued for long-term infection and pain control or can be discontinued if the drainage and pain has ceased, with the ability to restart the regimen if symptoms and/or signs of infection return.

NOTE! It is important to inform the patient and to include in the written prescription to take amoxicillin or doxycycline on an empty stomach for best absorption. It is also necessary to relate that doxycycline should be taken with clear liquids and to avoid milk and dairy products for 1 hour before and 1 hour after taking the capsule. This is due to the fact that dairy products bind tetracyclines like doxycycline, preventing gut absorption. Also, when prescribing metronidazole, instruct the patient to discontinue or limit alcohol use.

Surgical management of DIONJ in the osteopenia/osteoporosis patient

The purpose and outcome of nonsurgical management is to control secondary infection and therefore pain as well as to limit the progression and extent of the DIONJ. Once this has been accomplished, the patient may choose to live with the exposed bone if their function is not impaired, thereby avoiding surgery. In up to 50% of cases, a drug holiday of 9 months or more from a bisphosphonate and 7 months or more from denosumab results in an exfoliation of the necrotic bone. This is due to a return of osteoclasts and their ability to resorb an involucrum between the necrotic and viable bone so that it will slough off on its own. Once this occurs,

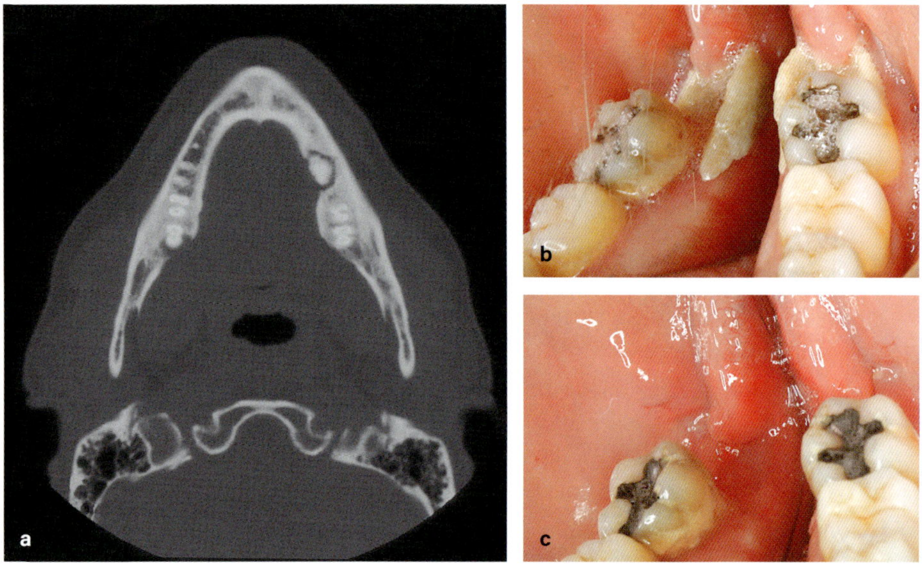

FIG 2-19 *(a)* Involucrum developing around necrotic bone that may cause mobility of the necrotic bone, spontaneous slough, or easy removal with a limited surgery. *(b)* Exposed bone from DIONJ. *(c)* Area of exposed bone seen in *b*, now healed after spontaneous slough during a drug holiday.

The purpose and outcome of nonsurgical management is to control secondary infection and therefore pain as well as to limit the progression and extent of the DIONJ.

the underlying granulation tissue matures and epithelializes to heal the area (Fig 2-19).

In cases where the amount of necrotic bone is too great to be resorbed or exfoliated, a surgery to remove all the necrotic bone becomes necessary. Once the appropriate drug holiday for either the bisphosphonate or denosumab is reached, a surgery can be planned to resolve the DIONJ. In the author's experience, the four most common types of curative surgery required for the osteopenia/osteoporosis patient with DIONJ are the following:

1. Removal of a portion of the lingual cortex of the mandible

During the drug holiday, an involucrum will form, but it may be incomplete. If the exposed bone is soft or somewhat mobile, it lends itself to a straightforward removal of the necrotic bone as a sequestrectomy via a lingual flap and a primary closure (Fig 2-20). This can be accomplished under local anesthesia or local anesthesia with IV sedation. The placement of platelet-rich plasma (PRP) or a bone marrow aspirate may also be used to enhance the healing of the bone and lingual flap.

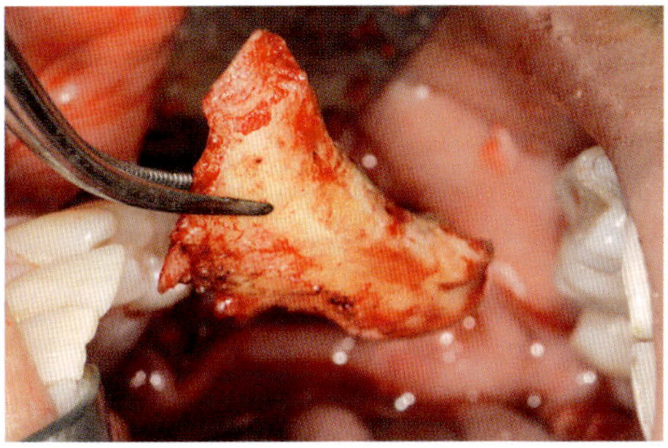

FIG 2-20 Removal of necrotic lingual cortex that became mobile due to a drug holiday.

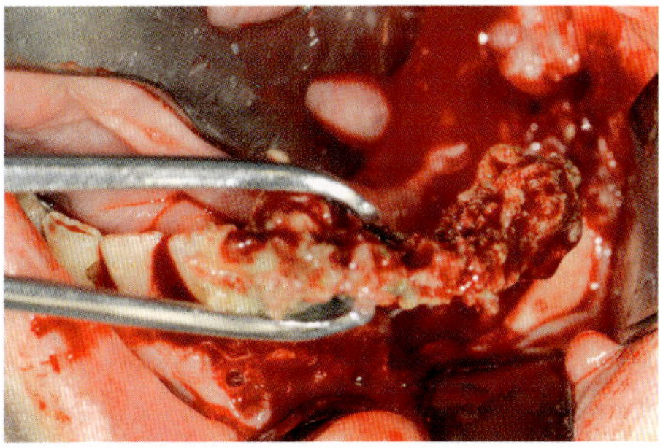

FIG 2-21 Extensive alveolar bone exposure removed via alveolectomy after a drug holiday.

2. Alveolectomy

Often the necrotic bone is from the extraction sockets of one or more teeth. In such cases, the drug holiday may form an involucrum between the necrotic alveolar bone and the underlying basilar bone. If the exposed bone is mobile, it will lend itself to a local sequestrectomy that also can be performed under local anesthesia or local anesthesia with IV sedation. If the exposed bone is not mobile and there is either an incomplete involucrum or none exists, then an alveolectomy is required, which usually requires an operating room–based surgery (Fig 2-21). In this case, the addition of PRP or a bone marrow aspirate is also suggested as an added benefit. Furthermore, the loss of gingiva and oral mucosa may require extensive undermining to gain a primary closure.

3. Maxillary sinus debridement with a buccal fat pad reconstruction

After the posterior mandible, the posterior maxillary area below the maxillary sinus is the next most common area for DIONJ. If the necrotic bone is superficial within an extraction socket and radiographs show a well-pneumatized maxillary sinus, a straightforward sequestrectomy below the sinus floor should be curative. However, more commonly the necrotic bone includes the sinus floor and causes a chronic sinusitis diagnosed by a partially or completely radiopaque sinus seen radiographically (Figs 2-22a and 2-22b). In this presentation, the necrotic bone and any teeth within it are removed along with the sinus floor, making an entry into the maxillary sinus. This opening may need to be enlarged at times using a modification of a Caldwell Luc approach. Once all the necrotic bone is removed (Fig 2-22c), the surgeon must completely debride the maxillary sinus (Fig 2-22d). One may be surprised about the amount of mucoceles, polyps, granulation tissue, and necrotic sinus that is removed (Fig 2-22e). Nevertheless, it is necessary to remove it all. If the buccal fat pad has not already herniated into the wound, it can be accessed by incising the periosteum in the posterior maxillary vestibule. The buccal fat pad is advanced with a gentle pericapsular dissection. It is advised to keep the point of the dissecting hemostat facing away from the fat so as to avoid macerating this friable tissue. If one gently tractions the buccal fat pad forward, small adherent bands will come into view that can be sharply incised with a scissor. The buccal fat pad can then be mobilized as far anterior as the canine area (Fig 2-22f). The surgeon should place the buccal fat pad into the sinus at the sinus floor level and suture it to one or two bur holes placed into the lateral sinus wall and to the palatal mucosa (Fig 2-22g). This will keep it in place and prevent retraction of the tissue. To complete the surgery, it will be necessary to undermine the buccal mucosa (Fig 2-22h). This will allow it to be advanced so as to gain a two-layer closure of the oral-antral communication.

The buccal fat pad is well suited for closing a large oral-antral communication due to its robust blood supply from two branches of the internal maxillary artery and the fact that it contains a large number of stem/progenitor cells. Once this site heals, a radiograph will note a repneumatization of the maxillary sinus and observe the buccal fat pad as appearing on the floor of the sinus (Figs 2-23). At this time, a type of sinus elevation graft may be accomplished by elevating the buccal fat pad as one would elevate a sinus membrane and graft between the buccal fat pad and the oral mucosa.

4. Continuity resection of the mandible

In the author's experience, 14% of mandibular DIONJ cases in osteopenia/osteoporosis patients are Stage III with uncontrollable symptoms and/or sufficient extension to recommend a continuity resection. In contrast to mandibular resections for osteoradionecrosis, which most always require a soft tissue replacement, usually with a microvascular flap, few similar resections for DIONJ in the osteopenia/osteoporosis patient require soft tissue replacement. The dissection is usually from a transcutaneous approach. The periosteum can be retained; it is unaffected by DIONJ-causing drugs because periosteal cells are not coupled to osteoclast-mediated bone resorption and renewal as are marrow cells, which maintain medullary trabecular bone. The margins of the resection are based on the radiographic assessment. Generally, 1 cm from each margin of radiographically involved bone is a good starting point. The surgeon should keep in mind that the ramus is not a specific target of DIONJ-causing drugs and is only involved as an extension from the bone anterior to it. Therefore, when radiographically normal-appearing bone in the ramus is evident, it can be considered a safe margin (Fig 2-24). The surgeon should assess the bone edges of the resection for bleeding points and some residual viable bleeding marrow space. Observation of a completely mineralized marrow space should alert the surgeon to a possibly inadequate resection margin.

14% of mandibular DIONJ cases in osteopenia/osteoporosis patients are Stage III.

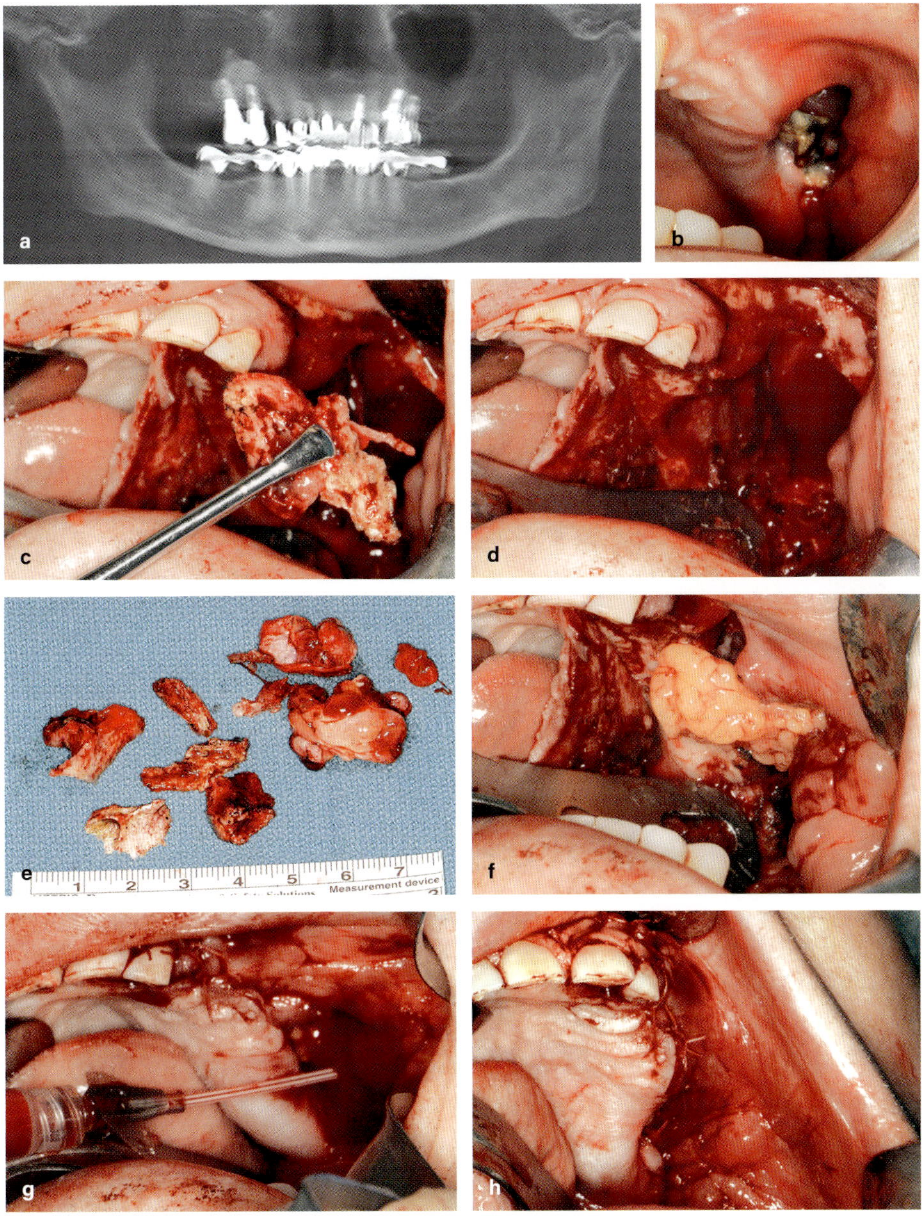

FIG 2-22 *(a and b)* Stage III DIONJ of the posterior maxillary alveolus and sinus floor producing a chronic sinusitis shown by opacification of the sinus airspace. *(c to e)* A large Caldwell Luc opening is necessary to remove the numerous mucoceles and infected sinus membrane in a DIONJ case involving the maxillary sinus. *(f)* Mobilizing and advancing the buccal fat pad to reconstruct the sinus floor assists in resolving the DIONJ and preventing an oral-antral communication. *(g)* Buccal fat pad positioned and stabilized into the floor of the sinus using sutures to adjacent uninvolved maxillary bone. Here PRP was added to the buccal fat pad. *(h)* Undermining the buccal mucosa for advancement over the buccal fat pad will achieve a two-layered closure.

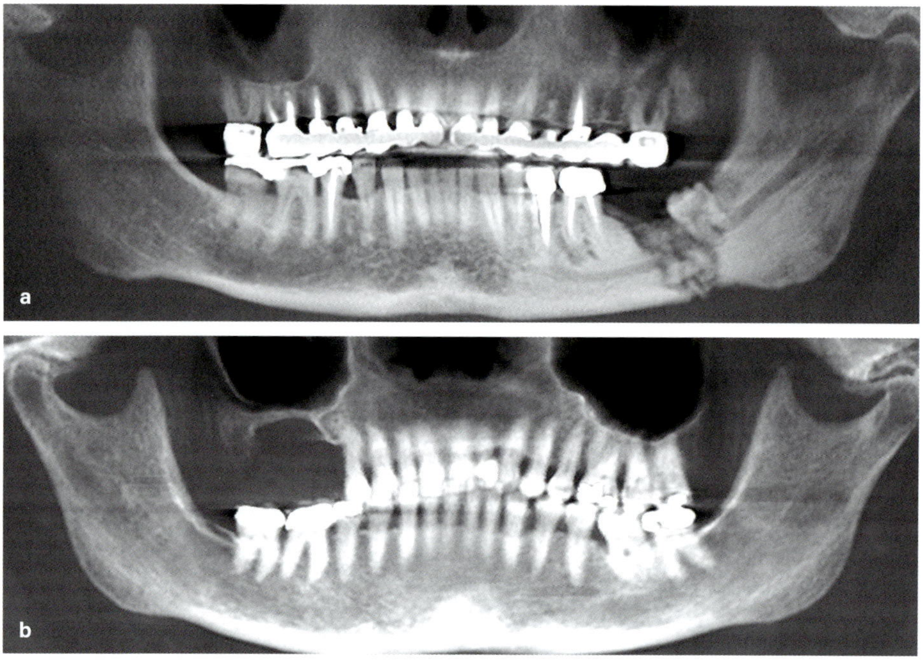

FIG 2-23 *(a)* Opaque right maxillary sinusitis due to DIONJ. Note the left maxillary and mandibular DIONJ. *(b)* A resolved DIONJ and resolved right maxillary sinusitis in a similar case noting a surgical defect in the maxilla and a completely repneumatized right maxillary sinus.

If there is sufficient soft tissue for coverage, a minimal amount of secondary infection, and resection margins that appear adequate, the surgeon may consider an immediate reconstruction. This can be accomplished with either an autogenous cancellous marrow graft or a tissue-engineered graft using cancellous allogeneic bone with recombinant human bone morphogenetic protein-2/acellular collagen sponge (rhBMP-2/ACS; 1 mg/cm of defect) and either PRP or a bone marrow aspirate (2 mL/cm defect; Fig 2-25). As an alternative, a free vascular osseocutaneous flap of fibula, iliac crest, or scapula may be used (Fig 2-26).

In cases where the bone is actively infected, it is best to accomplish the resection and debridement of any infected soft tissue and defer bone grafting.

In cases where the bone is actively infected, it is best to accomplish the resection and debridement of any infected soft tissue and defer bone grafting. In such cases, the placement of a 3-mm-thick titanium plate as an "artificial jaw" may be used to retain mandibular continuity and support the patient's nutritional requirements as well as appearance until the tissue has healed sufficiently to support a bone graft (Fig 2-27).

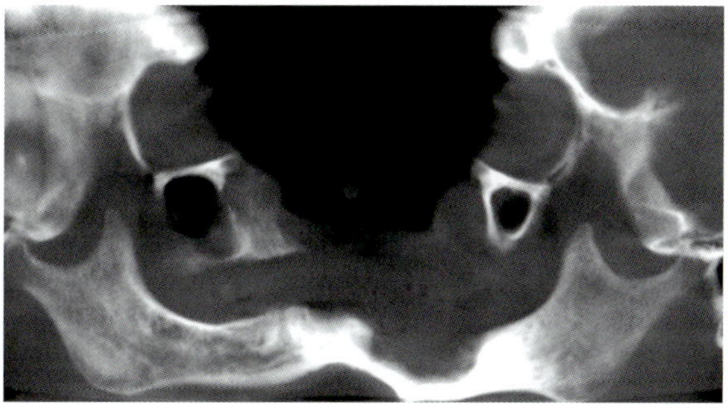

FIG 2-24 If radiographic signs of DIONJ are absent in the ramus, it implies a resection margin in healthy bone.

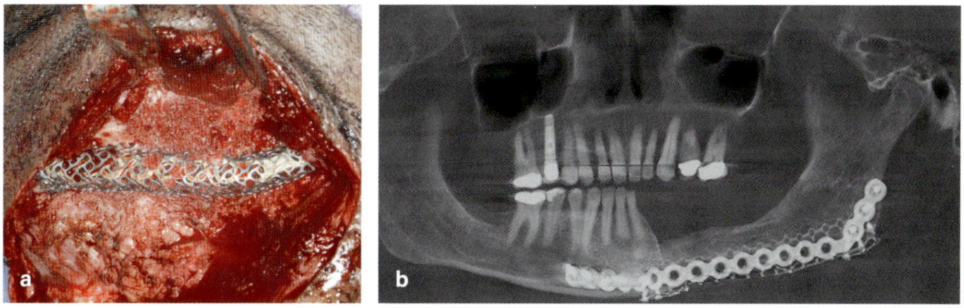

FIG 2-25 *(a)* In the noncancer patient, rhBMP-2/ACS combined with cancellous allogeneic bone and either PRP or bone marrow aspirate afford a reconstruction with low morbidity. *(b)* Bone regeneration in a resection for DIONJ using PRP, rhBMP-2/ACS, and cancellous allogeneic bone.

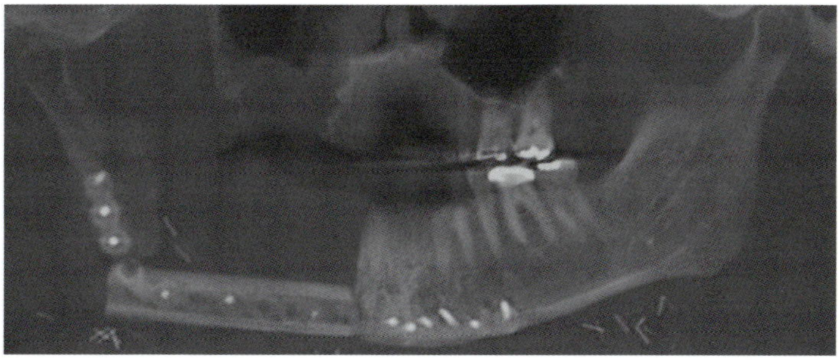

FIG 2-26 In selected cancer patients or those with significant soft tissue loss, a free vascular osseocutaneous flap offers a means of reconstructing defects resultant from DIONJ.

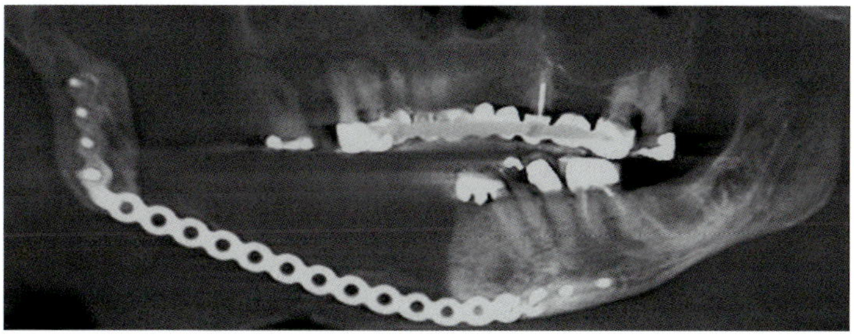

FIG 2-27 In such cases where a biologic reconstruction is not advised, a titanium reconstruction plate is used to gain continuity in the concept of an artificial jaw.

Sample Cases

Case 1 — A 55-year-old woman with postmenopausal osteoporosis

Patient evaluation

- **Chief complaint:** "I need implants. My dentist doesn't want to do them because of my medication."
- **History of present illness:** Diagnosed with osteoporosis 1 year ago. She was started on alendronate 70 mg/wk 9 months ago.
- **Previous medical history:** No known major comorbidities; no known allergies.
- **Oral examination:** Missing mandibular teeth nos. 18, 19, 20 and maxillary teeth nos. 13, 14, 15; no exposed bone.
- **Radiographic examination:** Adequate height and width of mandibular ridge for dental implants; hyperpneumatized maxillary sinus with insufficient bone for implants.

Suggested course of action

1. Treatment plan for dental implants in the mandible and sinus elevation bone graft in the maxilla.
2. Request a 3-month drug holiday from the treating physician.
3. Provide the treating physician with a list of alternative drugs with no risk or DIONJ (ie, calcium plus vitamin D3, raloxifene, teriparatide, abaloparatide, strontium renelate, strontium citrate).
4. Proceed with treatment plan as soon as drug holiday is begun.

Rationale

Although the recommended drug holiday for a patient taking alendronate would be 9 months prior to the surgery and 3 months after, this person has taken alendronate for less than the 2 years that would create a significant DIONJ risk. Therefore, in this case the procedures can be accomplished once the drug holiday has begun, and alendronate can be restarted 3 months later. This is sufficient time for the sinus elevation, bone graft, and the implant osseointegration to be well on its way to maturity.

Case 2	A 62-year-old woman with postmenopausal osteoporosis

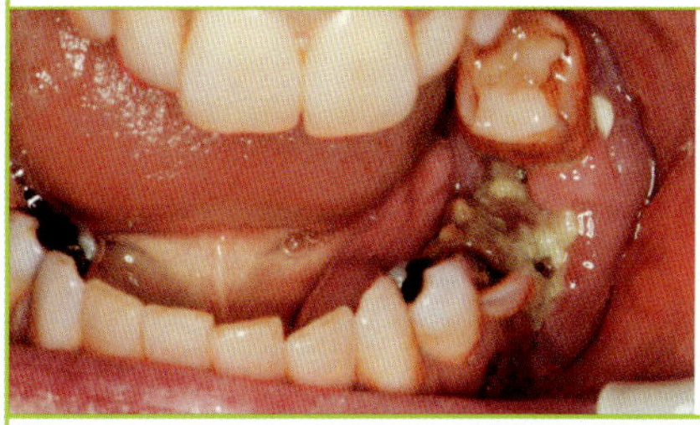

Patient evaluation

- **Chief complaint:** "My bridge came off and now there are only roots left."
- **History of present illness:** Diagnosed with osteoporosis 2 years ago. She has never taken bisphosphonates but has been on denosumab 60 mg every 6 months subcutaneous for 2 years, the last dose 2 months ago.
- **Previous medical history:** No known allergies; mild hypertension for which she takes amlodipine 5 mg/day and hydrochlorothiazide 12.5 mg/day.
- **Oral examination:** Residual roots of teeth nos. 28, 29, and 31 with root caries. There is no evidence of infection and no exposed bone.
- **Radiographic examination:** Normal trabecular bone pattern; no obvious osteosclerosis or osteolysis.

Suggested course of action

1. Treatment plan the removal of the residual roots with the option for immediate dental implants if desired or socket grafting.
2. Defer surgery until the patient has been off denosumab for 4 months (another 2 months).
3. Because of the need for a 4-month denosumab-free period (ie, drug holiday), request that the prescribing physician delay the next scheduled denosumab injection by 1 month so as to gain a 3-month healing period.

Rationale

As a RANK ligand inhibitor that affects bone marrow osteoclast precursors as well as peripheral adult osteoclasts, patients are at risk after just two doses of denosumab. The short half-life of denosumab allows for a 4-month drug holiday to reduce the risk to negligible. This patient was already effectively 2 months into a drug holiday. Therefore, a 2-month delay before removing the residual roots provides maximal risk aversion and offers the possibility for socket grafting or immediate dental implant placement.

Case 3 — A 47-year-old woman is referred to you by her oncologist to evaluate abscessed teeth.

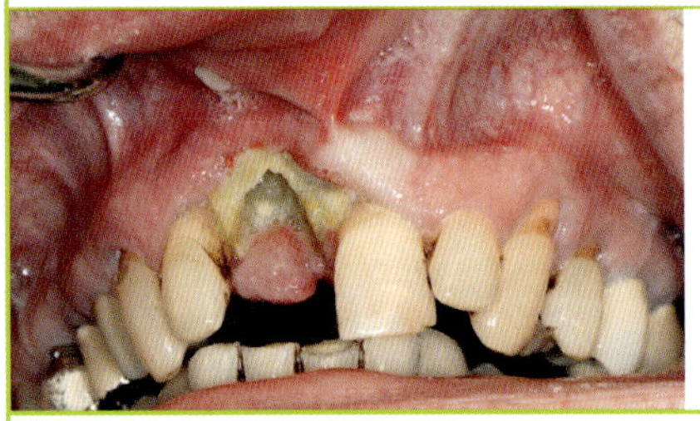

Patient evaluation

- **Chief complaint:** "I have exposed bone and pain coming from my upper teeth."
- **History of present illness:** Toothaches and abscesses have continued for years. Now, several chronically neglected teeth are abscessing. The oncologist ordered a morning fasting serum CTX test. The result was 310 pg/mL.
- **Previous medical history:** Diagnosed with breast cancer 3 years ago. There is no evidence of metastasis, comorbidities, or known drug allergies.
- **Medications:** Letrozole and Faslodex (AstraZeneca) for her maintenance chemotherapy. Alendronate 70 mg/wk since the diagnosis for breast cancer to prevent drug-induced osteoporosis from letrozole. The mandible is edentulous.
- **Radiographic examination:** Maxillary anterior six teeth have bone with evidence of osteolysis.

Suggested course of action

1. Treatment plan to remove the maxillary anterior six teeth, debride necrotic bone, irrigate thoroughly, smooth sharp areas of bone, gain a primary closure, and provide a provisional prosthesis. Accomplish this treatment plan after a 9-month drug holiday.
2. Disregard the CTX in this case because of the cancer diagnosis.
3. Request an alendronate drug holiday of 9 months from the oncologist. Provide a list of alternative drugs that can be used to prevent osteoporosis without risking DIONJ (ie, calcium plus vitamin D3, raloxifene, teriparatide, abaloparatide, strontium renelate, strontium citrate). Also, inform the patient and the oncologist that neither Faslodex nor letrozole pose a risk for DIONJ and can be safely continued.
4. Palliate pain and control infection with amoxicillin 500 mg TID ongoing throughout the drug holiday and metronidazole 500 mg TID for a limited 10-day course initially and backup prescription to be added to the ongoing amoxicillin if an acute flare-up infection develops.
5. Incise and drain any acute abscess cavities and culture the contents.
6. Remove abscessed teeth and debride infection once the 9-month drug holiday has been achieved.
7. Continue the drug holiday for 3 months after the surgery. →

Case 3 (cont)

Rationale

While a CTX of 310 pg/mL would usually indicate that the surgery could be performed with little or no risk for DIONJ, the cancer makes this test invalid. The CTX measures a fragment of collagen cleaved off by the osteoclast as it resorbs bone. Therefore, it is a good measure of systemic osteoclast function. However, cancers split off collagen fragments that cross-react with the CTX test to register a falsely high number. Therefore, in this case, one must rely on the proven efficacy of the drug holiday.

The amoxicillin-metronidazole combination initially is designed to control the dentoalveolar infection quickly and therefore reduce the pain. The ongoing amoxicillin is designed to maintain control of the infection throughout the drug holiday so that when the extraction and the debridement is performed, the bacterial load is minimal.

Case 4 | A 64-year-old postmenopausal woman

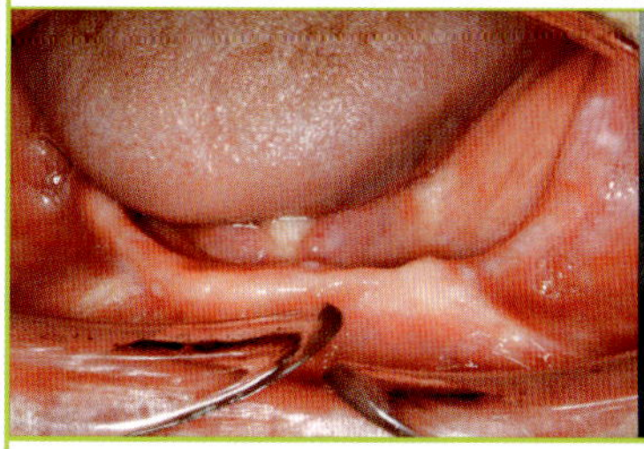
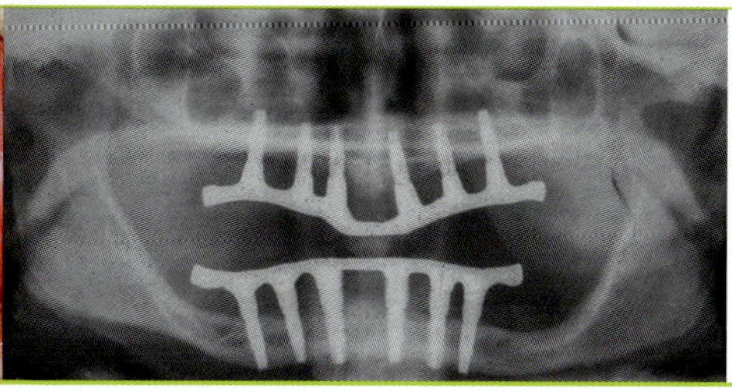

Patient evaluation

- **Chief complaint:** "I can't keep my lower denture in. I need implants."
- **History of present illness:** A long-time edentulous patient with a relatively small mandible has a well-fitting retentive maxillary denture but an ill-fitting and mobile mandibular denture.
- **Previous medical history:** Rheumatoid arthritis for 20 years, under good control; otherwise no other medical conditions. Took prednisone 40 mg/day in the past but currently at 10 g/day. Took methotrexate 2.5 mg/day in the past but is now off of that medication. Took alendronate 70 mg/wk for 8 years but has not taken it for the past 18 months. The rheumatologist ordered a morning fasting serum CTX test with the result of 97 pg/mL. →

Case 4 (cont)

- **Oral examination:** There is an edentulous mandibular ridge in a Class III position to the maxilla. There is no exposed bone. Slight bilateral lower lip hypoesthesia presumably due to denture compression on the mental nerves.
- **Radiographic examination:** A CBCT measures the edentulous ridge to be 11 mm in average height and adequate width. There are no areas of osteolysis or osteosclerosis. There is an incidental finding of bilateral condylar head erosion and flattening unassociated with any symptoms. The mental foramen has been displaced to the second molar area due to the alveolar bone resorption.

Suggested course of action

Treatment plan for an implant-retained mandibular denture using a modified "All-on-4" concept. Disregard the CTX in this case due to the history of prednisone and methotrexate.

Because the patient has already been off alendronate for 18 months (an adequate drug holiday), the procedure can be performed at this time.

Rationale

While a CTX of only 97 pg/mL would normally indicate a high risk for DIONJ, the history of even prednisone alone or methotrexate alone invalidates the test. This is due to the fact that the CTX measures a collagen fragment split off from bone as osteoclasts resorb bone and is thus an index of systemic osteoclast activity. However, because glucocorticoids deplete the amount of collagen in bone, the amount of collagen fragments released by osteoclasts normally resorbing bone of this type is less. This results in a falsely low number. In addition, methotrexate inhibits the functionality of osteoclast precursors, which in turn liberate fewer collagen fragments as osteoclasts resorb bone, once again resulting in a falsely low number.

Despite a relatively small mandible and the negative effect of a past history of alendronate, prednisone, and methotrexate, this patient remains a reasonably good candidate for dental implants. An 11-mm mandibular height is sufficient to place 10-mm implants without a risk of fracture if the implants are placed 1 cm apart. Because this patient has been on an extended drug holiday from alendronate and because the bone into which the implants are to be placed is basilar bone and not alveolar bone, the risk of DIONJ is maximally reduced.

The modification of the "All-on-4" concept suggested here takes advantage of the posteriorly displaced mental foramen. In this case, the angled implant can be placed in the second premolar area and should be placed more upright to balance the occlusal load more evenly.

Case 5 A 68-year-old postmenopausal woman

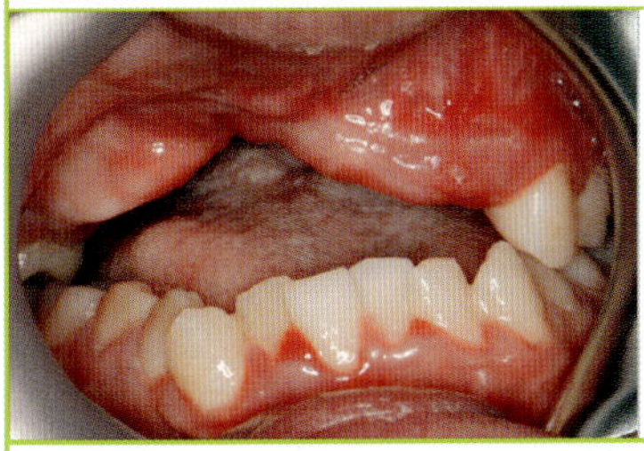

Patient evaluation

- **Chief complaint:** "I fell down yesterday and cut my chin. I also loosened several lower front teeth. The emergency room said I was okay but that I needed to see a dentist."
- **History of present illness:** This lady tripped and fell on her chin, resulting in a chin laceration and dental injuries. The chin laceration was sutured. She was placed on cephalexin 500 mg QID.
- **Previous medical history:** She has been on alendronate 70 mg/wk for 2 years. She has no comorbidities and no known allergies. A CTX test among others were taken in the emergency room last night. All were within normal limits including the CTX at 212 pg/dL.
- **Oral examination:** Tooth no. 25 was completely avulsed but remains in its socket with an attached fragment of buccal bone. Teeth nos. 24, 25, 26, and 27 are 2+ to 3+ mobile, but the sockets of these teeth are intact. The remaining mandibular dentition is intact with occlusal restorations in molars. The gingiva and oral mucosa are edematous and congested. The tissue bleeds on probing.
- **Radiographic examination:** Periapical radiographs indicate minimal damage to the alveolar bone except in the area of tooth no. 25, in which the alveolus is lost and is apparently attached to the avulsed tooth no. 25.

Suggested course of action

1. Repeat the CTX so that it is taken as a morning fasting blood draw.
2. Take a panoramic radiograph or CBCT scan to rule out condylar fractures.
3. Remove tooth no. 25. Replace teeth nos. 24, 26, and 27 in their sockets and splint them together and to posterior teeth.
4. Suture or Coe-Pack dress the gingiva into position around the teeth.
5. Change the antibiotic to amoxicillin 500 mg TID for 10 days along with metronidazole 500 mg TID for 10 days.
6. Inform the prescribing physician of the injury and your treatment. Request a 3-month drug holiday from alendronate and send the list of osteoporosis-effective drugs with no risk for DIONJ as an alternative to alendronate.
7. Maintain splinting long-term (ie, 6 months) unless complications arise. →

Case 5 (cont)

Rationale

The assessment of a fracture, particularly a condylar fracture, is a standard of care issue. Because, in this case, the emergency room didn't recognize the potential for a condylar fracture, the responsibility falls on the dental practitioner.

A completely avulsed tooth and bone complex portends a poor prognosis. However, mobility of teeth from an injury with a minimally traumatized alveolus has a reasonably good prognosis.

Oral injuries of bone and soft tissue involving the periodontal area must use antibiotics with a spectrum that includes anaerobes. Cephalexin has poor sensitivity against anaerobes. Therefore, amoxicillin and metronidazole is a better choice when several teeth have been lost should an infection develop.

The CTX taken in the emergency was unreliable due to it not being a morning blood draw. However, acute injuries such as this do not allow for a drug holiday, and necessary treatment must be rendered accepting a DIONJ risk. In this case, the morning fasting serum CTX test was returned as 225 pg/dL, giving reassurance that DIONJ was unlikely and illustrating that validity of the CTX test is relevant in situations when a drug holiday cannot be undertaken and when the test is not corrupted by cancer, glucocorticoids, or methotrexate.

Case 6 — An 80-year-old woman with postmenopausal osteoporosis

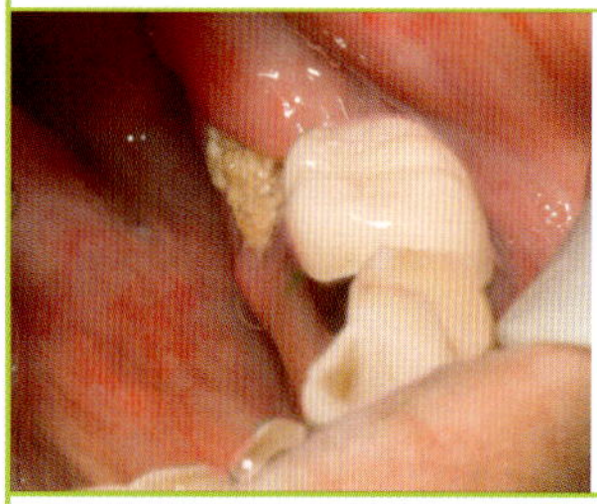

Patient evaluation

- **Chief complaint:** "I have bone coming through my gums."
- **History of present illness:** This woman initially took raloxifene followed by risedronate and is now taking alendronate 70 mg/wk for osteoporosis. Her T-scores have not improved greatly during 15 years of treatment. Her last T-score was –2.9. She says her physician is contemplating switching to denosumab.
- **Previous medical history:** Type II diabetes, hypertension, and hypercholesterolemia are all well controlled. She reports an allergy to penicillin that causes "throat swelling."

Case 6 (cont)

- **Medications:** Amlodipine, metformin, Lipitor (Viatris)
- **Oral examination:** There is a 2 cm × 1 cm area of exposed bone in the left posterior lingual area. The bone is immobile and nontender. There is no drainage noted. It is located lingual to tooth no. 18 and extends to the retromolar area. Her occlusion is centric, but the wear pattern on the crown on tooth no. 18 implies a premature contact.
- **Radiographic examination:** A diffuse increase in mineralization is noted around the molar area. The surface of the exposed bone is noted to be irregular and mottled. No osteolysis or involucrum is seen.

Suggested course of action

1. Explain to the patient that the cause of the exposed bone is most likely the alendronate and that the exposed bone is not painful now because it is not infected but that it can become painful if it does become infected.
2. Examine the occlusion with articulation paper. Relieve any areas of excessive occlusal loading, especially on teeth in the area of the exposed bone.
3. Treat with 0.12% chlorhexidine oral rinses twice daily. Provide a backup prescription for doxycycline 100 mg/day to begin only if pain develops and schedule for a surveillance appointment in 4 months or sooner if pain or drainage develops.
4. Request a drug holiday of 9 months from the prescribing physician and send them the list of alternative drugs not known to cause DIONJ. It is also suggested to warn the physician that the dental profession has noted a rapid extension and worsening of DIONJ if denosumab is prescribed after a patient has already been taking a bisphosphonate.

Rationale

- Well-controlled type II diabetes, hypertension, and hypercholesterolemia are not sufficiently severe comorbidities to significantly alter DIONJ treatment.
- Repetitive occlusal overloading requires a faster and more intense remodeling mediated by osteoclasts. Relieving traumatic occlusion will work toward reducing the amount of exposed bone and the severity of the DIONJ.
- The 0.12% chlorhexidine is designed to reduce the oral microbial colonization of the exposed bone to prevent it from becoming infected and therefore painful. The backup prescription of doxycycline is used due to the penicillin allergy, and the patient is instructed to use it only if an infection develops.
- The drug holiday is designed to allow the bone marrow to repopulate the diminished osteoclast population so that an involucrum can begin and a sequestration process can occur. If the exposed bone sloughs off during the drug holiday, the mucosa will cover the underlying bone. If the bone becomes mobile or if repeated infections develop during the drug holiday, a surgical debridement (sequestrectomy) via a lingual flap should be considered.

Case 7 | A 77-year-old postmenopausal woman

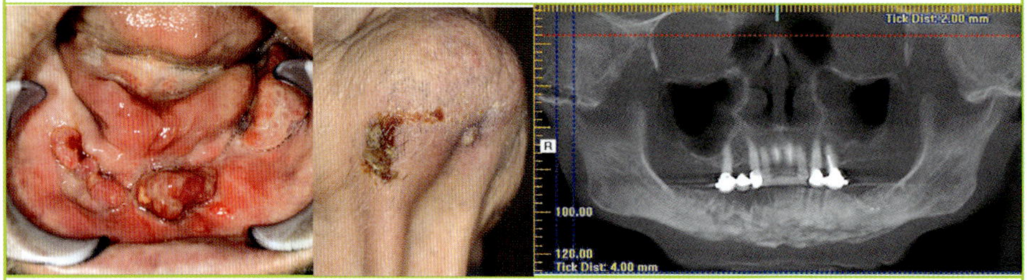

Patient evaluation

- **Chief complaint:** "I have bone coming through my gums and it hurts more and more every day."
- **History of present illness:** This woman took alendronate 70 mg/wk for 4 years to treat osteoporosis. When her T-scores failed to improve, she was switched to denosumab. After just two doses of denosumab, exposed bone and pain developed in the mandible. She has now received two additional doses of denosumab for a total of four doses. She is scheduled for another dose this month. Her prescribing physician has referred her to you.
- **Previous medical history:** Osteoporosis, age-related cataracts, hypercholesterolemia, gout, gastroesophageal reflux disease. She reports no known allergies.
- **Medications:** Prilosec (Procter & Gamble), allopurinol, indomethacin
- **Oral examination:** There is a nearly complete exposure of the lingual plate on each side of the mandible, including the midline area. There is a slight seropurulent exudate that can be expressed with the elicitation of pain upon palpation. The remaining maxillary dentition is stable but has 1+ mobility. There are also draining fistulas at the inferior border in the right parasymphysis and midline areas.
- **Radiographic examination:** A CBCT scan shows an incomplete involucrum of the lingual cortex bilaterally. In the right parasymphysis area, a tract of osteolysis is seen extending into the inferior border.

Suggested course of action

1. As initial treatment, splint the maxillary anterior teeth and prescribe amoxicillin 500 mg TID for an unlimited time and metronidazole 500 mg TID for a limit of 10 days.
2. Alert the prescribing physician that your diagnosis is Stage III DIONJ and that a pathologic fracture is threatened. →

Case 7 (cont)

3. Request that the prescribing physician begin a 9-month drug holiday from both alendronate and denosumab and send them the list of alternative medications for osteoporosis that have no risk for DIONJ.
4. Plan for an inpatient surgery to remove the lingual plate exposed bone and curette the tract of osteolysis as well as excise the cutaneous fistula. It is also recommended to place either a section of rhBMP-2/ACS between the lingual flap and the medullary bone surface or PRP or a bone marrow aspirate to enhance the healing potential.

Rationale

- This more advanced-stage presentation of DIONJ is frequently seen when a bisphosphonate (alendronate) is changed to a RANK ligand inhibitor (denosumab).
- Initial therapy to control infection and stabilize the dentition works toward limiting the extension of the DIONJ and promotes a faster resolution of infection after the sequestrectomy.
- The gout medications this patient was taking have no negative effects on facial bones and do not require discontinuation.
- Placement of the rhBMP-2/ACS sponge between the lingual flap and the exposed medullary bone of the mandible after removing the sequestrum will enhance the soft tissue healing via its property of upregulating vascular endothelial growth factor (VEGF) and its fundamental effect of proliferation and differentiation of osteoprogenitor cells. PRP and/or a bone marrow aspirate work in a similar fashion.
- The immediate to early surgery is made possible by the fact that the alendronate was last taken before the four doses of denosumab, which was 2 years ago and therefore well within the 9-month drug holiday benchmark. The last dose of denosumab was apparently 5 months earlier, which is within the 4-month drug holiday recommended for denosumab.

Case 8 A 71-year-old postmenopausal woman

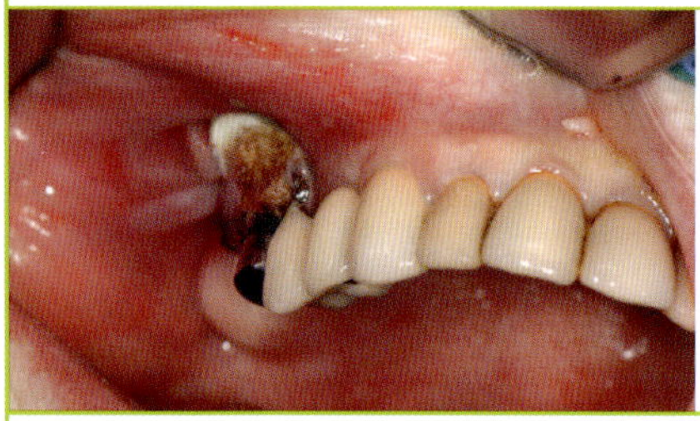

Patient evaluation

- **Chief complaint:** "My tooth socket hasn't healed and it's been 3 months. Now I can't even breathe out of the right side of my nose."
- **History of present illness:** This woman preferred the convenience of a once per year injection for her osteoporosis treatment over taking the oral medication alendronate that required 16 oz of water and an upright posture for 1 hour. Therefore, she was started on zoledronate 5 mg IV once per year. She has been receiving zoledronate yearly for the past 6 years and received her last dose 6 months ago.
- **Previous medical history:** No significant medical conditions. No known drug allergies. She currently only takes vitamin supplements.
- **Oral examination:** Exposed bone in the socket of tooth no. 3. Teeth nos. 1 and 2 are missing. There is a slight seropurulent drainage coming from the tooth socket. The remainder of the occlusion is stable with no mobility.
- **Radiographic examination:** There is a combination of osteolysis and osteosclerosis in the alveolar bone above the socket of tooth no. 3 as well as the maxillary sinus floor. The airspace of the right maxillary sinus is entirely radiopaque. The left maxillary sinus is fully pneumatized. No other pathologies are noted.

Suggested course of action

1. Begin initial treatment by prescribing amoxicillin 500 mg po TID and 0.12% chlorhexidine mouth rinses.
2. Defer surgery for 3 months so as to reach a 9-month drug holiday.
3. Inform the patient and the prescribing physician that zoledronate was the cause of the DIONJ and that the regular dosing schedule of once per year can be resumed in 6 months. However, note that continued zoledronate IV places her at risk for a recurrence or a new site of DIONJ. Forward the physician the list indicating the hierarchy of osteoporosis drugs related to their risk for DIONJ.

Case 8 (cont)

4. After 3 months, accomplish an inpatient surgery to remove the necrotic bone in the socket of tooth no. 3 and likely tooth no. 4 as well as the maxillary sinus floor. Make a Caldwell Luc entry into the maxillary sinus and extensively debride the mucoceles, polyps, and inflamed/necrotic membrane. Culture tissue taken from the sinus and submit for histopathology. Contour any sharp areas of bone and place two bur holes in the lateral sinus wall above and anterior to the Caldwell Luc entry. Incise the periosteum in the posterior lateral portion of the vestibule to access the buccal fat pad. Using a pericapsular blunt dissection with the point of the hemostat directed away from the buccal fat pad assisted by gentle traction, advance the buccal fat pad forward and place it into the maxillary sinus. Suture the buccal fat pad to the palatal mucosa and suspend it forward by suturing it to the bur holes placed in the lateral maxillary wall. Undermine the buccal flap to gain a closure over the buccal fat pad, thereby gaining a two-layered closure.

Rationale

- DIONJ involving the maxillary sinus floor frequently causes an extensive chronic sinusitis that will persist as long as necrotic bone exists. Amoxicillin is a first-line drug for maxillary sinusitis.
- Because IV zoledronate is given once per year, the 9-month drug holiday fits into the protocol if the dental team accomplishes the needed surgery 9 months after the last dose and 3 months before the next dose.
- The surgeon should not be hesitant to remove the entire sinus lining and the contents of the sinus. Residual necrotic tissue in the sinus will result in a recurrent chronic sinusitis. The healthy sinus will regenerate a new sinus membrane and will become repneumatized.
- A culture of the tissue will assist in any antibiotic changes if the infection persists.
- The buccal fat pad has a rich blood supply and numerous progenitor cells. This accounts for a success rate of this procedure of over 95%. It gains a two-layer closure and can be part of a sinus elevation graft if accomplished once the healing is complete.

Case 9 A 69-year-old postmenopausal woman

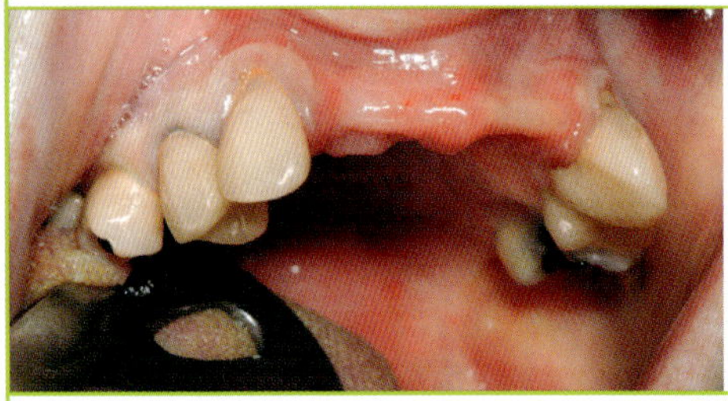

Patient evaluation

- **Chief complaint:** "My dentist says I need implants but won't do them because of my osteoporosis medications."
- **History of present illness:** Diagnosed with severe osteoporosis 3 years ago due to a T-score of –3.8 and two vertebral fractures; she was started on alendronate for 2 years. Because the alendronate failed to improve her T-scores, she was switched to teriparatide. She has now taken two of the three 28-day cycles of teriparatide 20 mcg sc daily.
- **Previous medical history:** Anxiety, Hashimoto's thyroiditis, restless leg syndrome
- **Medications:** Synthroid (AbbVie), Celexa (Allergan), gabapentin
- **Oral examination:** Partially edentulous jaws with adequate bone for implant-supported bridges in the mandible but a knife-edge ridge in the anterior maxilla
- **Radiographic examination:** The CBCT scan confirms the oral examination findings. Of particular note, the knife-edge maxillary ridge has an adequate vertical height to accommodate 11.5-mm implants but has a thin residual buccal plate of only 2 mm.

Suggested course of action

1. Treatment plan for and proceed with indicated implants in the mandible and a horizontal ridge augmentation graft in the maxilla. Consider using PRP or bone marrow aspirate together with rhBMP-2/ACS to augment and enhance the bone formation in the graft.
2. Inform the prescribing physician of your treatment plan and that there is no contraindication to continue with teriparatide, adding that teriparatide actually assists your graft procedure and the osseointegration of the implants.
3. Allow at least 6 months for graft maturity before placing implants and the same time frame for complete osseointegration of the implants. →

Case 9 (cont)

Rationale

- Because this patient has been on a drug holiday from alendronate for at least 1 year, that drug is already beyond the recommended 9-month drug holiday and is of no significant concern for the treatment plan.
- Teriparatide is FDA approved specifically for "severe osteoporosis." Its mechanism of action is a stimulation of osteoblasts and therefore focuses its benefit on regenerating new elastic bone rather than retaining old excessively mineralized and brittle bone, as do bisphosphonates and RANK ligand inhibitors. Therefore, teriparatide will assist the bone formation of the maxillary graft and the osseointegration of the implants.
- The full 6-month protocol for graft maturity and osseointegration is necessary. Although osteoporosis is diagnosed from T-scores derived from DEXA scans of the pelvis (hip), vertebrae (spine), and wrists, osteoporosis is a systemic skeletal disease that also involves the mandible and maxilla. This makes the bone-to-metal contact in dental implants less than that in those without osteoporosis and reduces the rate and degree of bone regeneration. Therefore, the use of PRP or a bone marrow aspirate and rhBMP-2/ACS are useful adjuncts in such patients.

Case 10 A 75-year-old postmenopausal woman

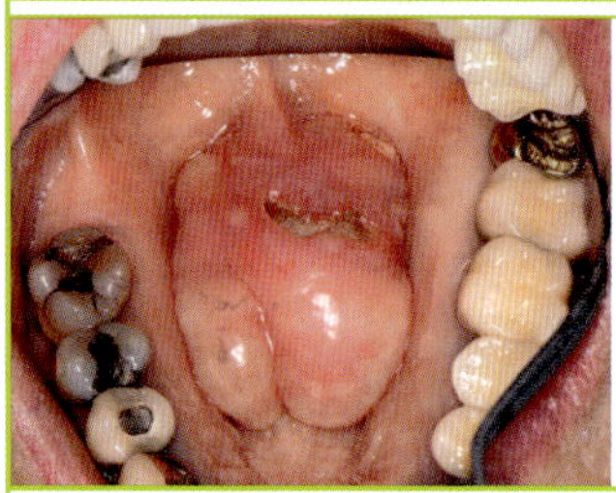

Patient evaluation

- **Chief complaint:** "The bone at the roof of my mouth is brown and painful. The pain runs up behind my eyes."
- **History of present illness:** This woman was diagnosed with osteoporosis 6 years ago and was placed on denosumab 60 mg every 6 months at that time, equating to 12 doses total. Her last dose was 1 month ago. Her pain has been steady since the bone became exposed after eating some hard chips that abraded the mucosa. Her only treatment has been clindamycin 300 mg TID, which was discontinued due to a pseudomembranous colitis requiring an emergency room admission and treatment with metronidazole, fluids, and electrolyte replacement.
- **Previous medical history:** Emphysema, chronic bronchitis, iron deficiency anemia, alcoholism, a continued smoking habit, type II diabetes. She reports no known allergies.
- **Medications:** Jardiance (Boehringer Ingelheim), albuterol, Spiriva (Boehringer Ingelheim), and ferrous sulfate
- **Oral examination:** There is a bilobulated midline maxillary torus that is represented by a brown discolored bone. The exposed bone is slightly mobile and is painful to touch. The surrounding palatal mucosa is somewhat edematous and boggy. There is a slight purulent exudate at the edge of the exposed bone to the mucosa.
- **Radiographic examination:** A CBCT scan shows an irregular surface of the torus but also osteolysis within the center of the torus and osteolysis extending anteriorly and posteriorly onto the palatal shelf. Both maxillary sinuses are well pneumatized.

Suggested course of action

1. Begin initial treatment with amoxicillin 500 mg TID ongoing together with metronidazole 500 mg TID limited to 10 days as well as 0.12% chlorhexidine oral rinses TID.
2. Treatment plan for an inpatient sequestrectomy of the torus and likely a portion of the palatal shelf together with a palatal push-back flap for coverage. →

Case 10 (cont)

3. Inform the prescribing physician of your plan for surgery in 2 months so as to gain a 4-month drug holiday from denosumab and the need to defer restarting denosumab for 1 month past the usual schedule to accommodate healing. Also, request a "medical clearance" for surgery under general anesthesia.
4. Take a maxillary impression to fabricate an acrylic cover splint of the palate to support the palatal flap.
5. Inform the patient about the increased general risks of surgery and general anesthesia due to her several comorbidities. Also inform the patient of a risk for an oral-nasal fistula that may require a second surgery or an obturator.
6. Placing PRP or a bone marrow aspirate on the oral side of the nasal mucosa is advised to enhance healing, as this tissue may be inflamed and friable. The palatal flap should be fully mobilized to approximate and close the midline defect and should also be suspended to any interproximal gingiva that is available. The oral splint is best relieved significantly and soft tissue relined before inserting it. Transdental wires should be used for retention as opposed to attempts at a palatal screw. Plan to leave this splint in place for 3 to 4 weeks.

Rationale

- The antibiotic coverage and the 0.12% chlorhexidine is designed to control the secondary infection, relieve pain, and prevent further extension of the DIONJ.
- The medical clearance and informed consent about surgical and anesthetic risks are required due to her comorbidities, especially her pulmonary insufficiencies.
- The surgery itself will be a challenging one. In many cases, the torus itself develops an involucrum, separating it from the palatal shelf. In such cases, the torus can be cleaved off the palatal shelf, which is viable, and granulates over in the next month or two. In this case, where scans show an osteolytic involvement of the palatal shelf into the nose, one should approach the anterior area between the piriform buttresses with a vestibular incision. In this approach, one can elevate the nasal mucosa off the nasal floor above the torus and insert a cotton pad soaked in phenylephrine as a guard. Therefore, when the palatal flap is developed, the necrotic bone can be removed with direct vision and delivered without violating the nasal mucosa and entering into the nasal cavity.

References

1. Anastrozole (Arimidex). https://www.medicinenet.com/anastrozole-oral/article.htm. Accessed 3 March 2021.
2. Letrozole. https://www.drugs.com/cdi/letrozole.html. Accessed 3 March 2021.
3. Santen RJ, Brodie H, Simpson ER, Siiteri PK, Brodie A. History of aromatase: Saga of an important biological mediator and therapeutic target. Endocr Rev 2009;30:343–375.
4. Marx RE, Cillo JE Jr, Ulloa JJ. Oral bisphosphonate-induced osteonecrosis: Risk factors, prediction of risk using serum CTX testing, prevention, and treatment. J Oral Maxillofac Surg 2007;65:2397–2410.
5. Kunchur R, Need A, Hughes T, Goss A. Clinical investigation of C-terminal cross-linking telopeptide test in prevention and management of bisphosphonate-associated osteonecrosis of the jaws. J Oral Maxillofac Surg 2009;67:1167–1173.
6. Kwon YD, Kim DY, Ohe JY, Yoo JY, Walter C. Correlation between serum C-terminal cross-linking telopeptide of type I collagen and staging of oral bisphosphonate-related osteonecrosis of the jaws. J Oral Maxillofac Surg 2009;67:2644–2648.
7. Leahey AM, Friedman DL, Bunin NJ. Bone marrow transplantation in pediatric patients with therapy-related myelodysplasia and leukemia. Bone Marrow Transplant 1999;23:21–25.
8. Black DM, Schwartz AV, Ensrud KE, et al; FLEX Research Group. Effects of continuing or stopping alendronate after 5 years of treatment: The Fracture Intervention Trial Long-term Extension (FLEX): A randomized trial. JAMA 2006;296:2927–2938.
9. Naik NH, Russo TA. Bisphosphonate-related osteonecrosis of the jaw: The role of *Actinomyces*. Clin Infect Dis 2009;49:1729–1732.

Chapter 3

Prevention and Management of DIONJ in Cancer Patients Taking Drugs Known to Cause DIONJ

While there are certainly similarities between the osteopenia/osteoporosis patient and the cancer patient who develops DIONJ, there are significant differences that must be understood.

What Are the Differences Between Osteoporosis Patients and Cancer Patients?

- In cancer patients receiving a bisphosphonate, the drug is infused intravenously. Therefore, their bone contains a higher concentration of the bisphosphonate.
- Cancer patients receiving denosumab receive it at twice the dose of osteoporosis patients.
- Denosumab is administered at six times the frequency in cancer patients as compared to osteopenia/osteoporosis patients.
- Cancer patients may also be treated simultaneously with antiangiogenic drugs, which will add to the DIONJ.
- Some cancer patients may develop DIONJ from an antiangiogenic drug alone (eg, bevacizumab, sunitinib).
- Cancer patients often have a greater number of and more significant comorbidities.
- The DIONJ in cancer patients is usually more extensive, requiring surgical interventions more frequently.
- The surgical interventions in cancer patients with DIONJ are usually more extensive and resective in design, with reconstruction options limited.

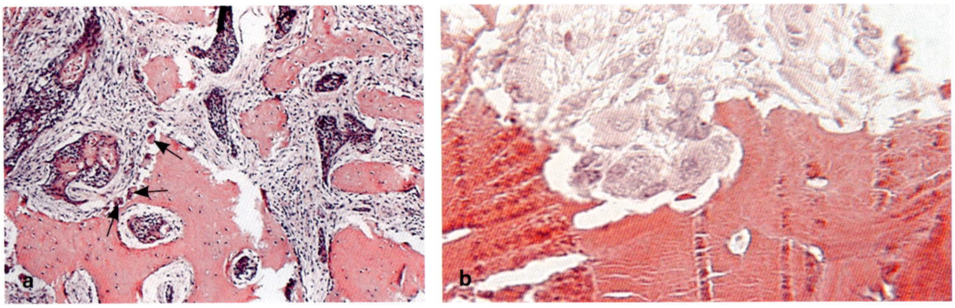

FIG 3-1 *(a)* Squamous cell carcinoma causes bone resorption not directly but mediated through osteoclasts *(arrows)*. *(b)* Pale and distended osteoclast dying from the toxic effect of a bisphosphonate.

How Do These Drugs Affect Cancer and also Cause DIONJ?

Bisphosphonates

Even though many cancers invade and resorb bone directly or metastasize to bone via resorbing a cavity in the bone, very few cancers have the internal enzymatic machinery to resorb bone by themselves. Instead, they resorb bone by recruiting osteoclasts to do it for them and then grow into the resorbed bone cavity (Fig 3-1a). This is done by their ability to secrete RANK ligand or a RANK ligand–like protein that locally activates the osteoclast to rapidly resorb bone.

The original drug used to prevent fractures from metastatic cancer and reverse any hypercalcemia of malignancy was pamidronate, administered intravenously at a dosage of 90 mg per month. This drug is now used sparingly, mostly because it requires a 90-minute infusion time. It has since been replaced by zoledronate at 4 mg per month. Zoledronate is two to five times more potent than pamidronate and is infused over just 15 minutes. It is twice as potent as oral alendronate, and because it is infused intravenously, it loads bone 140 times faster and more completely, making IV zoledronate at 4 mg/month a very high risk for DIONJ.[1]

The bisphosphonate class of drugs act as cellular poisons by irreversibly inhibiting the enzyme farnesyl synthase.[2] Therefore, as the cancer-stimulated osteoclast begins to resorb bone that is loaded with a bisphosphonate, it literally ingests the bisphosphonate, which kills the osteoclast in less than 24 hours and thus halts the bone resorption.[2] This action is microscopically documented by observing a ballooning of the osteoclast with fragmentation of its many nuclei and final cellular bursting (Fig 3-1b). This antiosteoclastic action reduces the weakening of bone and therefore the risk for pathologic fractures from cancer-directed resorption. It also prevents the release of calcium into the bloodstream, thus reversing hypercalcemia. However, it is this same antiosteoclastic action that reduces alveolar bone remodeling and renewal, which in turn causes DIONJ and midshaft femur fractures.

Denosumab

Denosumab drugs are direct inhibitors of RANK ligand and are therefore also antiosteoclastic drugs.[3] While they kill osteoclasts as they resorb bone, the main action of denosumab is to deplete their numbers by inhibiting their development and to neutralize the action of RANK ligand produced by the cancer.[4] Therefore, despite the cancer signaling the osteoclast to resorb bone for its spread, there are few or no osteoclasts to respond to the signal. Because denosumab has a more profound effect on developing osteoclasts than bisphosphonates do, it is a major cause of DIONJ, equal to or even more so than zoledronate.

Because denosumab has a more profound effect on developing osteoclasts than bisphosphonates do, it is a major cause of DIONJ, equal to or even more so than zoledronate.

Antiangiogenic drugs

The antiangiogenic drugs known to cause DIONJ by themselves are bevacizumab and sunitinib. From the initial work of Judah Folkman,[5,6] it has been long realized that cancers recruit blood vessels to themselves for their growth and metastasis. Therefore, the concept of limiting the recruitment of nutrient blood vessels to the cancer (choking it off) is attractive and was initially thought to be the cure for all cancers (the magic bullet). However, most cancers mutate to develop alternative angiogenic stimuli, relegating today's antiangiogenic drugs to be only adjuncts and part of a chemotherapy drug protocol utilizing several drugs.

Bevacizumab is specifically used in lung cancer patients with and without metastasis.[7] It is a direct potent inhibitor of vascular endothelial growth factor (VEGF).[8] By eliminating VEGF and therefore its nutrient supply, lung cancers grow more slowly and can be contained to a degree. In repetitive dosing, its reduction of blood supply to the alveolar bone can result in necrotic bone, particularly in the face of one of the initiating factors referred to in chapter 1. Sunitinib is a very potent inhibitor of several growth factors including VEGF.[9] It is a common drug used together with others in the treatment protocols for renal cancers and gastrointestinal stromal tumors with or without metastasis.[10] Similarly to bevacizumab, repetitive dosing can result in necrotic alveolar bone via reduced blood flow, particularly if combined with any of the initiating factors discussed in chapter 1.

The Three Phases of Prevention and Management of DIONJ in Cancer Patients

The role of the dental professional in the management of cancer patients taking drugs known to cause DIONJ is to support these patients faced with this life-threatening disease and to support the oncologist's efforts. The perspective to keep in mind is that runaway cancer is life-threatening. While DIONJ may be painful and cause dysfunction, it is not usually life-threatening. Therefore, the goal in preventing and managing DIONJ in cancer patients is pain control, infection control, reduction in inflammation, and/or resolution where possible so that the oncologist can continue their cancer treatment without breaks in the schedule or events that would result in halting their treatment altogether.

The perspective to keep in mind is that runaway cancer is life-threatening. While DIONJ may be painful and cause dysfunction, it is not usually life-threatening.

Phase I: Preventive Measures Before Starting a Drug Known to Cause DIONJ

One of the great services the dental professional can provide to cancer patients is to develop a working relationship with oncologists. When an oncologist recognizes a cancer metastasis to bone or seeks to prevent one by using a drug known to cause DIONJ, they do not usually need to begin treatment immediately. Therefore, the dental team has an opportunity to reduce the risk for DIONJ by improving the dental health of the patient. It is reasonable to request that the oncologist defer the use of bisphosphonates or denosumab for 2 months in order to accomplish necessary oral care. Even then, the risk for zoledronate does not become significant until four doses, and for pamidronate eight doses, allowing the dental team at least 3 months' time to eliminate potential initiating factors. Because denosumab kills osteoclasts faster by its direct effects on their development, its risk becomes significant with the second dose, so the dental team has only 1 month beyond any deferment of starting denosumab. The time to develop a significant DIONJ risk from bevacizumab and sunitinib is less well known. However, because cases from these drugs have mostly occurred with repeated doses, a 2-month period before starting these drugs is reasonable.

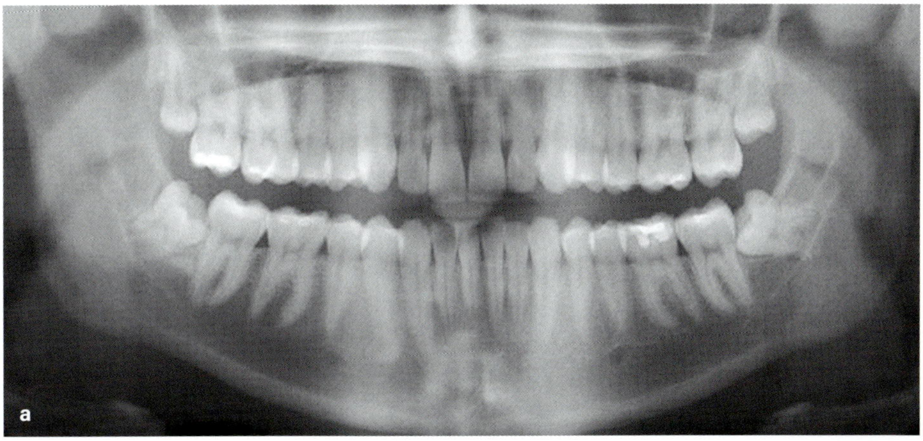
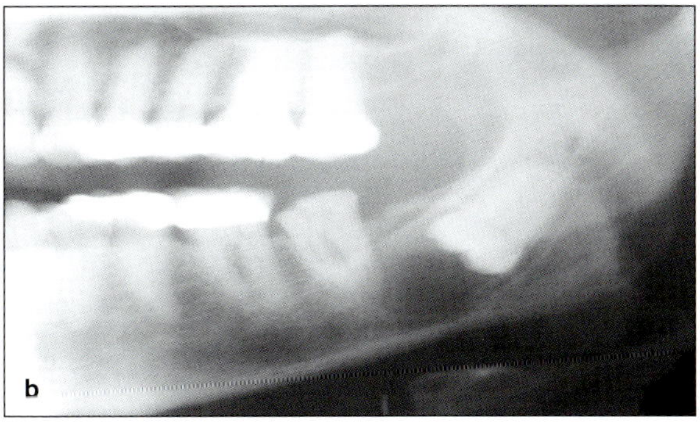

FIG 3-2 *(a)* Soft tissue and partial bony impacted third molars should be considered for removal before starting a drug known to cause DIONJ. *(b)* Complete bony impactions without associated pathology are best left to remain.

What should be done prior to the patient starting on a drug known to cause DIONJ?

1. Remove nonrestorable teeth and periodontally hopeless teeth

Because extraction is the most frequent initiating factor for DIONJ, removing these teeth prior to the commencement of the drug will prevent the need for extraction while the patient is actively taking the drug and thereby prevent the initiation of DIONJ. One should also consider removing soft tissue and partial bony impacted third molars in which part of the crown is erupted, creating the possibility of pericoronitis (Fig 3-2a). However, complete bony impactions or those fully covered by soft tissue that have no associated pathology are best left in place (Fig 3-2b).

2. Eliminate periodontal inflammation via either surgery or deep scaling

Because DIONJ always starts in the alveolar bone, ongoing inflammation that increases the need for bone resorption and remodeling will either initiate DIONJ by itself or result in the need to extract the involved tooth or teeth.

3. Dental prophylaxis and serious oral hygiene instruction by a dental hygienist

Because chemotherapy causes mucositis and nausea, cancer patients receiving chemotherapy often have significant plaque accumulation due to their reluctance to brush and floss. This can lead to inflammation, periodontal bone loss, and the need to remove teeth while the patient is actively taking a DIONJ-causing drug. In no other patients are frequent dental prophylaxis and oral hygiene instructions more required or important, as their chemotherapy treatments are most often long-term over several years.

4. Occlusal adjustments and splint therapy for bruxism and/or mobile teeth

Repetitive occlusal overloading from a premature contact, a crown with a premature contact, or a dental implant with a heavy contact traumatizes the alveolar bone, requiring an increased rate of bone turnover and often resulting in direct injury. The author has noted numerous DIONJ cases directly linked to occlusal trauma as the initiating factor. Therefore, balancing the occlusion for an even contact across the arches is recommended, as is splint therapy for patients suspected to be bruxers or those who recognize their bruxing habit. Additionally, stabilizing mobile teeth that are not indicated for extraction via splint therapy also reduces the inflammation, alveolar bone injury, and the need for bone remodeling, which will reduce the potential for DIONJ.

5. Restore restorable teeth and control any caries

Restoring restorable teeth and eliminating caries prior to the cancer patient starting a DIONJ-causing drug prevents the need for removing teeth or the development of dental abscesses while actively receiving these drugs. Too often caries is left untreated in restorable teeth prior to cancer therapy, only to progress more rapidly during treatment due to the side effects of chemotherapy and cancer therapy–induced poor oral hygiene. The best time to complete needed restorations and caries control is prior to beginning chemotherapy.

The best time to complete needed restorations and caries control is prior to beginning chemotherapy.

Phase II: Managing the Patient Actively Taking a Drug Known to Cause DIONJ with No Exposed Bone

This group is at high risk for developing DIONJ and should be approached with a knowledge of the risks related to each drug, how long they have taken it, when the last dose was administered, and the comorbidities of each patient. The goal in these patients is to maintain the dentition and support ongoing oral health without initiating DIONJ so as to allow continued oncologic therapy. The following recommendations are designed to accomplish this goal:

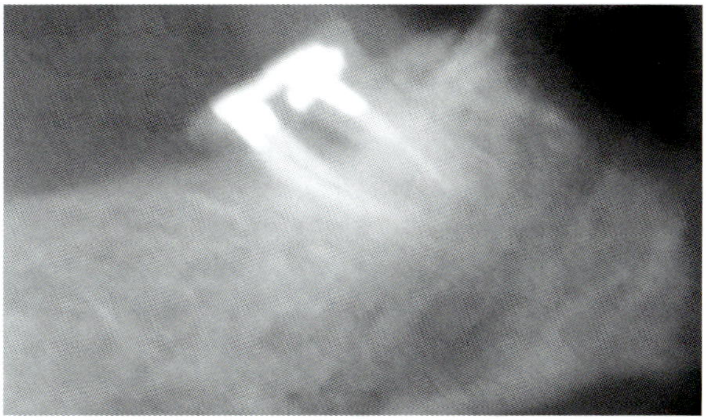

FIG 3-3 Root banking may be considered as an alternative to extraction in a patient at risk for DIONJ.

- **Avoid elective surgeries that may initiate DIONJ:** These include extractions, periodontal osseous surgery, crown lengthening, and dental implant placements. In the uncommon situation of unresolvable pain such as with a cracked tooth or abscessed tooth uncontrolled with root canal therapy and/or an incision and drainage procedure with antibiotics, an extraction may be unavoidable. In such situations, one should remove the tooth for pain relief, infection control, and to limit the local infection while giving the patient the warning and providing written informed consent as to a significant risk for DIONJ.
- **Treat all dental caries:** If the tooth is nonrestorable, consider root canal therapy and crown amputation (root banking) so as to avoid the open wound of an extraction socket (Fig 3-3). If the tooth is restorable, remove all caries and restore the tooth.
- **Maintain professional oral hygiene:** Perform dental prophylaxis every 3 months reinforcing good oral hygiene habits at each appointment.
- **Splint mobile teeth:** Splinting mobile teeth will reduce the increased rate of bone remodeling. Continued tooth mobility will predispose to DIONJ due to the reduction in osteoclasts required for bone remodeling/renewal around mobile teeth.
- **Maintain occlusal balance:** Maintain occlusal balance with occlusal equilibration as necessary and treat bruxism with splint therapy. This will also reduce the need for osteoclast-mediated bone remodeling/renewal.

Phase III: Managing the Patient with Exposed Bone from DIONJ

In these patients, it is critical to know the drug that was taken, if the patient was switched to another drug, how long they were taking each drug, and when the last dose was taken. The primary reason for this is that zoledronate's half-life of 11.2 years precludes the value of a drug holiday unless it is of 7 years or more. However, because denosumab is not bound to bone and has a half-life of only

26 days, a drug holiday has some usefulness even in cancer patients. Additionally, if the patient initially took zoledronate and was then switched to denosumab, this scenario predicts a more extensive and advanced stage of DIONJ. Therefore, a hierarchy of more advanced stage of DIONJ with greater symptoms and dysfunction follows in descending order:

Severity risk for DIONJ in cancer patients

- Zoledronate followed by denosumab
- Denosumab as a single drug
- Zoledronate as a single drug
- Pamidronate as a single drug
- Sunitinib as a single drug
- Bevacizumab as a single drug

It is useful to remind the oncology patient that only those drugs listed above are known to cause DIONJ and that their current chemotherapy drugs do not pose a risk for DIONJ and can continue.

Recommendations for treating patients presenting with exposed bone

It is useful to remind the oncology patient that only those drugs listed above are known to cause DIONJ and that their current chemotherapy drugs do not pose a risk for DIONJ and can continue. It is also useful to inform the patient that pain is the result of secondary infection, not the exposed bone itself. Inform the patient that your goal is to control pain and infections so that they can continue with their cancer therapy as well as to limit the spread and extension of the DIONJ. Furthermore, the patient may need to adapt to living with exposed bone if pain and infection can be controlled and their functional abilities maintained. Inform the patient that surgery may become necessary if the pain and infection cannot be controlled or if the DIONJ becomes sufficiently extensive as to threaten or create a functional disability related to eating, swallowing, or speech. The following recommendations are designed to achieve these goals:

1. Avoid office-based debridements requiring flap reflection in patients when pain and infection is controlled. While it is recommended to smooth sharp areas of exposed bone that abrade the tongue, many of us have learned that well-meaning local limited debridements are often counterproductive.

2. If the patient presents without pain, treat the exposed bone with 0.12% chlorhexidine oral rinses TID and prescribe a backup prescription of amoxicillin 500 mg TID to be used only if pain should develop. If the patient is allergic to penicillin, prescribe doxycycline 100 mg once daily as a substitute for amoxicillin and instruct the patient to avoid dairy products 1 hour before and 1 hour after talking the doxycycline for maximum absorption.
3. If the patient presents with pain, treat with 0.12% chlorhexidine oral rinses TID, amoxicillin 500 mg TID, and a limited 10-day course of metronidazole 500 mg TID. Instruct the patient to continue with the amoxicillin for 2 more weeks after the metronidazole. If the pain is resolved, the patient should continue with the 0.12% chlorhexidine oral rinses and only restart the amoxicillin if pain returns.
4. Inform the oncologist of your DIONJ diagnosis and relate to them that discontinuation of the causative drug is advisable. However, if their remains a therapeutic advantage for the patient to continue on the drug, there is no contraindication to continue it. Relate that you will continue to manage the oral health with these recommendations as well as those preventive measures outlined for those taking the drug with no exposed bone.
5. A reasonable follow-up protocol for DIONJ surveillance and adjustment of treatment is every 4 months or less if complications arise.
6. In patients with persistent pain and/or infection where radiographs identify localization of the necrotic bone to the alveolar process, torus, or lingual plate, a sequestrectomy of the involved bone should be considered.
7. Consider a major resection if:
    - Pain, infection, frequent bouts of swelling, and/or drainage occur and have been minimally responsive to antibiotics
    - A pathologic fracture occurs
    - A cutaneous fistula continues to drain while the patient takes antibiotics
    - A chronic maxillary sinusitis develops

NOTE! Many surgeries for DIONJ in the cancer patient will need to be performed without a drug holiday. However, those cases caused by denosumab alone will benefit from a drug holiday of 4 months or more due to its 26-day half-life. Also note that resections for cancer patients are done as a last option due in part to the fact that some patients are a poor anesthetic risk due to their very cancer and comorbidities but also due to the fact that reconstruction options are limited. That is, donor bone for either a cancellous marrow graft from the ilium or a free vascular fibula graft may transplant malignant cells. Additionally, rhBMP-2/ACS is contraindicated in patients with "exigent malignancies," which describes this patient population. Therefore, in a mandibular resection, a 3-mm-thick off-the-shelf titanium reconstruction plate or a cast virtual-planned titanium plate as an "artificial jaw" may be the only option.

Sample Cases

Case 1	A 58-year-old woman with known metastatic breast cancer is referred to evaluate her risk for DIONJ if teeth nos. 18 and 19 are removed and planned for a removable partial denture.

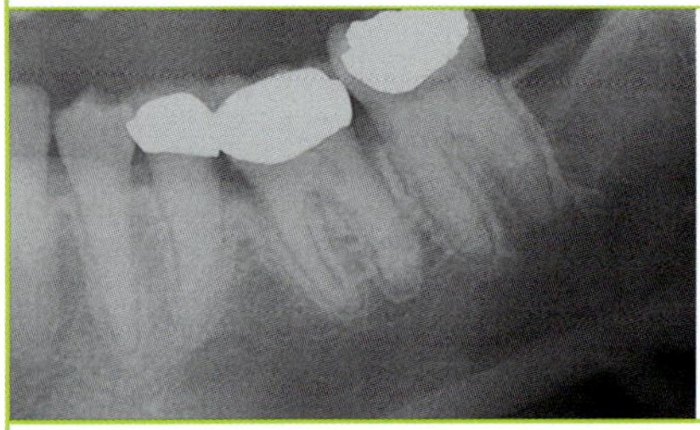

Patient evaluation

- **Chief complaint:** "My dentist says there is decay at the crown margins. I have no pain, and I eat well."
- **History of present illness:** Breast cancer diagnosed 10 years ago. Was NED (no evidence of disease) until 4 years ago when bony metastasis was noted in the scapula and pelvis. She has been on zoledronate 4 mg/month for 4 years and received the last dose 2 weeks ago.
- **Previous medical history:** No significant comorbidities. She is currently on Faslodex (AstraZeneca) maintenance.
- **Oral examination:** Crowns on teeth nos. 18 and 19. The dentition is in a good state of repair otherwise. No exposed bone. No significant periodontal inflammation.
- **Radiographic examination:** A significant sclerosis of the lamina dura is noted around all the roots of the posterior teeth bilaterally. There is also a slight increased mineralization of the alveolar bone.
- **Diagnosis:** Stage 0 DIONJ

Suggested course of action

1. Advise against extraction for teeth due to a high risk for clinical Stage I DIONJ.
2. Recommend patch restorations or crown replacements as opposed to extraction.
3. Consider root canal therapy for the molars in question if caries threatens or extends into the pulp.
4. Examine the occlusion carefully and accomplish occlusal equilibration if any teeth are in traumatic occlusion.
5. Inform the oncologist that the jaws show definitive signs of zoledronate toxicity and that if there is no further cancer benefit from zoledronate, it would reduce the risk for DIONJ if it is discontinued for now. Also relate that switching to denosumab will increase the risk for DIONJ. →

Case 1 (cont)

Rationale

- Zoledronate for 4 years places this patient in a high-risk category for DIONJ despite the absence of comorbidities.
- The sclerosis of the lamina dura involving several teeth represents Stage 0 DIONJ. If these molars are extracted, there is a high likelihood for nonhealing sockets and overt DIONJ. Therefore, alternative dentistry should be used to avoid the inherent initiation of DIONJ from extractions of teeth in this individual.
- The fundamental action of zoledronate is to eliminate osteoclastic bone remodeling and renewal. Therefore, it retains old bone that is hypermineralized. Because the lamina dura in the jaws remodels faster and more than the bone in other skeletal areas, it may become sclerotic and unable to remodel if the teeth are extracted, resulting in DIONJ.
- If zoledronate is discontinued, it may prevent the Stage 0 from progressing to Stage I or more.
- If denosumab replaces zoledronate, its strongly toxic effects on osteoclast precursors in the bone marrow have been known to add to and exacerbate the zoledronate effects, resulting in a rapid development of DIONJ.

Case 2

A 56-year-old man with metastatic prostate cancer is referred by his oncologist for a "dental clearance" prior to zoledronate therapy.

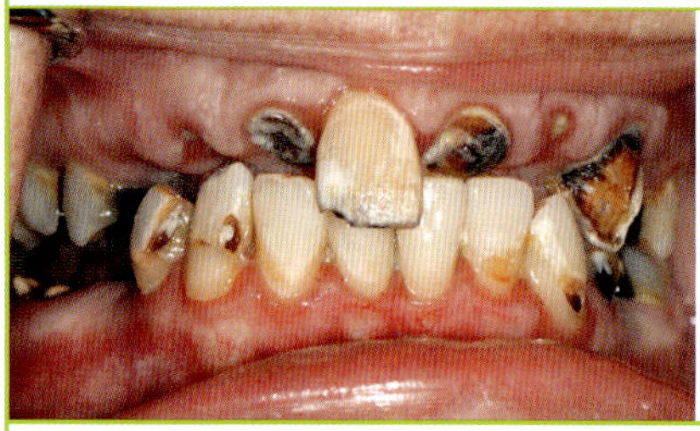

Patient evaluation

- **Chief complaint:** "I am here for my dental clearance."
- **History of present illness:** Diagnosed with prostate cancer 4 years ago with a Gleeson scale of 8. He was treated initially with radical prostatectomy and Lupron (AbbVie). A recent increase in his serum prostate-specific antigen (PSA) showed an increase from 1.8 to 24. A positron emission tomography (PET) scan noted vertebral and rib metastases.
- **Previous medical history:** No known allergies, and no other significant medical conditions
- **Oral examination:** Heavy plaque and calculus formation. Significant caries with residual roots from teeth nos. 5, 6, 7, 9, 10, 11, and 30. Moderate generalized periodontitis. No exposed bone, fistulas, or lymphadenopathy.
- **Radiographic examination:** A panoramic film shows small chronic periapical abscesses involving several teeth or residual roots. There is no evidence of osteolysis.

Suggested course of action

1. Contact the oncologist to request that they defer starting the zoledronate for 2 months. Explain that this patient is not "dentally cleared" but that after 2 months he should be able to begin zoledronate.
2. Because this patient seems to have neglected his teeth and oral health, the first step is to proceed with a thorough dental prophylaxis and oral hygiene instructions.
3. Remove residual roots and nonrestorable teeth. Contour the alveolar bone to eliminate sharp bony projections should partial dentures be fabricated.
4. Restore any restorable teeth with emphasis on crown coverage.
5. Refer the patient to a periodontist for evaluation and treatment of the periodontitis.
6. Relate to all dental specialists treating this patient to expedite their care so that the patient can begin zoledronate within 2 months.
7. Follow up with a removable partial denture to stabilize the occlusion. →

Case 2 (cont)

Rationale

- The goal is to accomplish the oral surgery and periodontal surgery procedures as soon as possible so as to gain a well-along healing process within 2 months.
- Because this patient is not in the habit of regular brushing and flossing or regular dental visits, dental prophylaxis is paramount early in the treatment course.
- Letting the oncologist know that you need to complete a significant amount of dental work before a "dental clearance" can be provided will reduce the chances of that doctor starting zoledronate too soon or switching to denosumab instead. It will also be appreciated by the oncologist, who may refer you additional patients.
- The removal of DIONJ-initiating factors at this time and stabilization of the occlusion will allow the oncologist to start and maintain zoledronate with a reduced risk of the patient developing DIONJ.
- A removable partial denture is recommended over dental implants due to the patient's upcoming zoledronate therapy as well as his track record of poor oral maintenance.

Case 3

A 62-year-old man is referred to you by another dentist because of exposed bone and exposed implants.

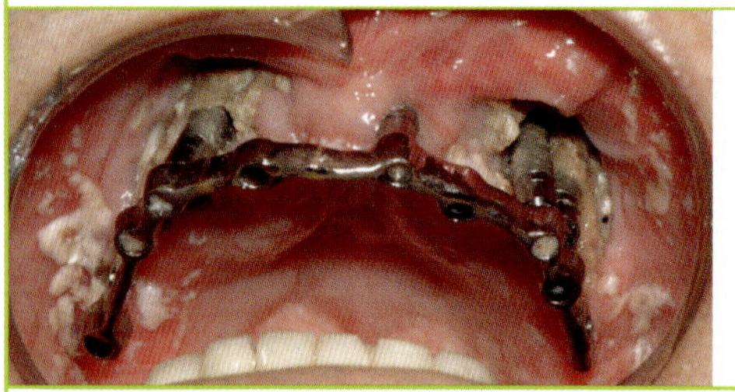

Patient evaluation

- **Chief complaint:** "My dentist wanted your opinion on this. He said I have an infection."
- **History of present illness:** This man has had a diagnosis of IGg long chain multiple myeloma for the past 2 years. He has previously undergone a stem cell transplant and several rounds of chemotherapy. He is considered in remission now and is on maintenance Revlimid (Celgene). He relates that the exposed bone has been present for 3 years and began 2 years after starting monthly zoledronate infusions.
- **Previous medical history:** Multiple myeloma–related anemia, hypertension, hypercholesterolemia, type 2 diabetes
- **Medications:** Zoledronate 4 mg IV monthly, Revlimid, Lipitor (Viatris), Metformin (Bristol-Myers Squibb), Losartan (Sandoz)
- **Oral examination:** There is evident exposed bone around the implants in the anterior maxilla. The implants are surprisingly clinically stable, and a screwed-in Hader bar is present that retains a clipped-on prosthesis. There is a slight sero-purulent exudate upon compression of the tissues around the exposed bone. The exposed bone is stable, as are the implants in the exposed bone. There are scattered areas of white soft patches that can be removed with a dental mirror.
- **Radiographic examination:** A CBCT scan shows mineralized bone around all the maxillary implants. There is some sclerosis but no osteolysis and no involucrum. The maxillary sinuses are well pneumatized bilaterally.
- **Diagnosis:** Stage II DIONJ

Suggested course of action

1. Prescribe nystatin oral suspension 100,000 units/mL; dispense two bottles of 473 mL each to be taken 2 tsp (10 mL) oral swish and spit three times daily to treat apparent candidiasis and because you will be likely to prescribe antibiotics.
2. Alert the oncologist of your Stage II DIONJ diagnosis and also of oral candidiasis, which may imply a reactivation of the multiple myeloma. →

Case 3 (cont)

3. Treat nonsurgically with amoxicillin 500 mg TID ongoing and metronidazole 500 mg TID for a limit of 10 days.
4. The patient may continue denture wearing for now despite the exposed bone around the implants.
5. Reevaluate the patient's response to the nystatin and the antibiotics in 2 weeks.

Rationale

- Multiple myeloma patients with DIONJ are the most difficult patients to manage due to the immune deficiency inherent in multiple myeloma.
- Candidiasis reflects either an alteration of the immune system or an imbalance in the normal oral flora from antibiotics. The oncologist will need to reexamine the multiple myeloma remission.
- It is not uncommon for multiple myeloma to be in remission for years and then suddenly exacerbate.
- An overview of this patient is one who is asymptomatic and functional with exposed bone. Therefore, controlling secondary infection while the oncologist evaluates the possible exacerbation of multiple myeloma is prudent.
- The goal of controlling infection and avoiding surgery that will seriously affect this patient's current function is the best approach at this time. Removing the necrotic bone and implants in the maxilla will negate his wearing a denture and commit him to complex reconstructive surgeries that are best avoided unless there is no other option.

Case 4

A 78-year-old woman with metastatic breast cancer is referred to you by her oncologist because of a "swollen jaw."

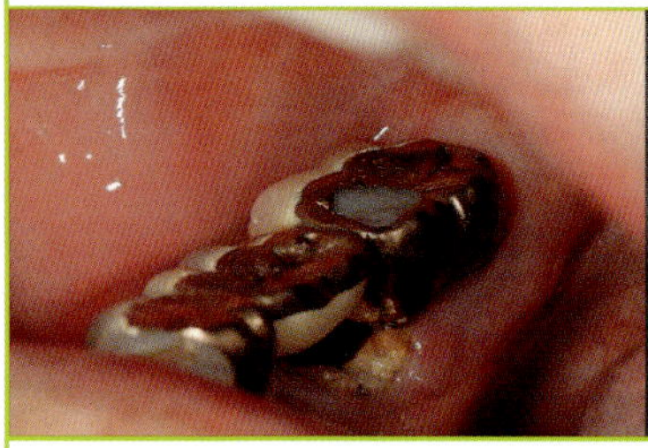

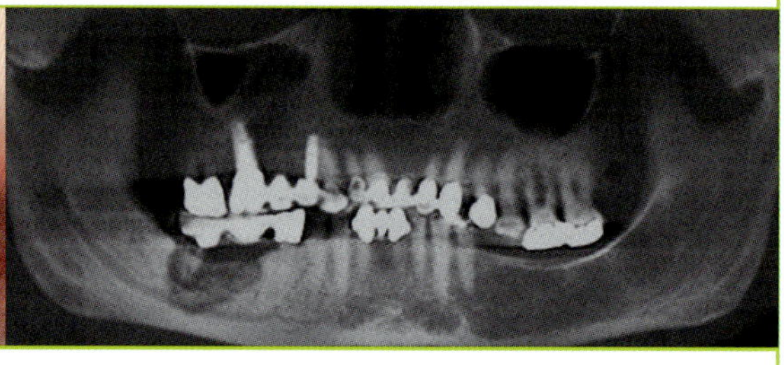

Patient evaluation

- **Chief complaint:** "My lower jaw began hurting last week. The swelling started 3 days ago."
- **History of present illness:** This woman was treated for breast cancer 12 years ago and was NED until 3 months ago when metastatic deposits were discovered in her humerus and ribs. She was started on denosumab 120/mg month subcutaneous 3 months ago. She has had two doses so far and is scheduled for her third dose later this week.
- **Previous medical history:** Breast cancer, glaucoma, cataracts, hypothyroidism, and a penicillin allergy causing "throat swelling"
- **Medications:** Timolol, Ibrance (Pfizer), Synthroid (Abbott)
- **Oral examination:** There is a 1 × 1 cm segment of exposed alveolar bone lingual to molar teeth nos. 29 and 31 and extending to bone under the pontic replacing tooth no. 30. The crowns on teeth nos. 29 and 31 have excessive wear. The contralateral side is missing mandibular molar and premolar teeth nos. 18, 19, and 20 with supraeruption of the opposing maxillary teeth. There is a slight purulent discharge around the exposed bone upon compression of the soft tissue. The remainder of the dentition is stable and well repaired.
- **Radiographic examination:** There is a significant osteolysis seen in the alveolar bone around tooth no. 31 and beneath the pontic in the no. 30 position. The opposing crowns in the maxillary arch represent the only posterior contact, as the teeth in the left maxillary arch are seen to be significantly supraerupted.
- **Diagnosis:** Stage I DIONJ

Suggested course of action

1. Prescribe doxycycline 100 mg/day ongoing and metronidazole 500 mg TID for a limit of 10 days as well as 0.12% chlorhexidine.
2. Alert the oncologist of your Stage I DIONJ diagnosis and request a 4-month drug holiday from denosumab. Relate that all other medications can continue including Ibrance. →

Case 4 (cont)

3. After a 4-month drug holiday, consider a transoral sequestrectomy and removal of teeth nos. 29 and 30 with undermining for a primary closure. Also consider removal of teeth nos. 13, 14, and 15 due to their extreme supraeruption and significant periodontal bone loss.
4. Once the surgical areas heal, consider removable partial dentures to achieve a bilateral balanced occlusion.
5. Continue the drug holiday from denosumab for another 3 months after surgery.

Rationale

- It is not unusual for breast cancer to first develop a metastasis many years after the patient has been "cancer free" without a recurrence at the original site.
- This case illustrates the very high potency of denosumab 120 mg/month and the significant initiation forces of traumatic occlusion to develop a rapid occurrence of DIONJ.
- Despite its use in a cancer patient with DIONJ, the short half-life of denosumab allowed for the effective use of a drug holiday to resolve this exposed bone short of a resection.
- The removal of the supraerupted maxillary teeth now takes advantage of the window of opportunity to reduce the potential for further problems once the denosumab continues as well as allows one to rehabilitate the patient to a stable occlusion with removable partial dentures.

Case 5 A 72-year-old woman with lung cancer

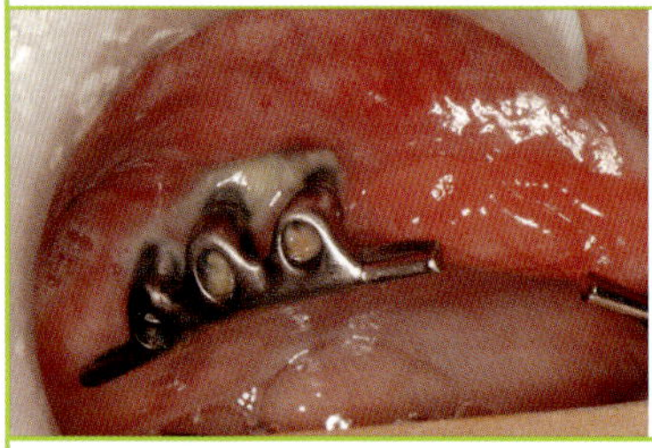

Patient evaluation

- **Chief complaint:** "The right side of my cheek is swollen and red."
- **History of present illness:** This woman was diagnosed with non–small cell lung cancer 3 years ago. She underwent a right lower lobe pneumonectomy 2 years ago. She was placed on chemotherapy including bevacizumab 500 mg every 2 weeks but developed bony metastasis 1 year ago, for which she began denosumab 120 mg/month. She has also been on nivolumab 240 mg every 2 weeks for the past 6 months. Her last denosumab injection was 2 months ago. She is scheduled for this month's injection later this week. Her swelling and pain began 2 weeks after her last injection of denosumab.
- **Previous medical history:** Former smoker (two packs a day) who quit 20 years ago. She has Hashimoto's thyroiditis and depression but reports no known allergies.
- **Medications:** Synthroid, Wellbutrin (GlaxoSmithKline), nivolumab 240 mg IV every 2 weeks, bevacizumab 500 mg every 2 weeks
- **Oral examination:** The maxilla is edentulous with three implants on each side retaining a maxillary full denture via separate Hader bars. On the right side, pus is draining around each of the implants, and exposed bone can be appreciated with probing around the implants. The oral mucosa is boggy in the area, and the right cheek is red and puffy. The implants are mobile and painful when palpated. There are no other areas of exposed bone or infection.
- **Radiographic examination:** There is significant osteolysis of the alveolar process and floor of the right maxillary sinus and complete opacification of the sinus airspace on the right. The left maxillary sinus is pneumatized, and the implants are within normal-appearing bone.
- **Diagnosis:** Stage III DIONJ

Case 5 (cont)

Suggested course of action

1. Prescribe amoxicillin 500 mg TID ongoing and metronidazole 500 mg TID for a limited 10-day course as well as 0.12% chlorhexidine oral rinses TID to gain control of the secondary infection.
2. Alert the oncologist of your diagnosis and request a drug holiday from denosumab for 2 more months before your planned surgery and 3 months thereafter for a total of 5 to 6 months. Relate that bevacizumab is also best postponed until 1 month after the surgery (a drug holiday of about 6 weeks). Also relate that all other medications including nivolumab can continue.
3. Once the drug holiday from denosumab has reached 4 months, accomplish a debridement surgery to remove the three implants and accomplish a radical sinus debridement known as a "radical sinusotomy" through a Caldwell Luc entry followed by irrigating the sinus with 0.12% chlorhexidine. As with a similar procedure outlined for DIONJ in an osteoporosis patient, access the buccal fat pad via an incision through the periosteum in the posterior maxillary vestibule. Advance the buccal fat pad into the sinus and suture it to transosseous bur holes placed through the lateral maxillary wall above the Caldwell Luc opening as well as to the palatal mucosa. The buccal mucosa is then undermined and advanced for a two-layer closure.
4. After the area heals, the denture can be reseated using only the residual Hader bar and a reline for retention.

Rationale

- A Caldwell Luc sinus debridement after a drug holiday has a very high success rate in the cancer patient population (just as it does in osteoporosis patients).
- This DIONJ was staged as Stage III due to the sinus extension.
- The rapid development of this Stage III DIONJ is mostly due to denosumab, but bevacizumab contributed to it significantly.
- Nivolumab is a monoclonal antibody against PDL-1 and is known as a "checkpoint inhibitor." It is prescribed mostly for lung cancer patients as well as more recently for oral/head and neck cancer, Hodgkin's lymphoma, and renal cancers. Nivolumab is not a drug known to cause DIONJ. It is effective in extending the life of these patients, but it is not a cure.
- Despite a partial pneumonectomy, patients such as this remain candidates for surgery under general anesthesia.
- The presence of the dental implants in this case was not likely to be contributory to the DIONJ any more than if natural teeth had been present. The potency and frequency of the two DIONJ-causing drugs were the likely cause.

Case 6 — A 52-year-old woman with metastatic breast cancer

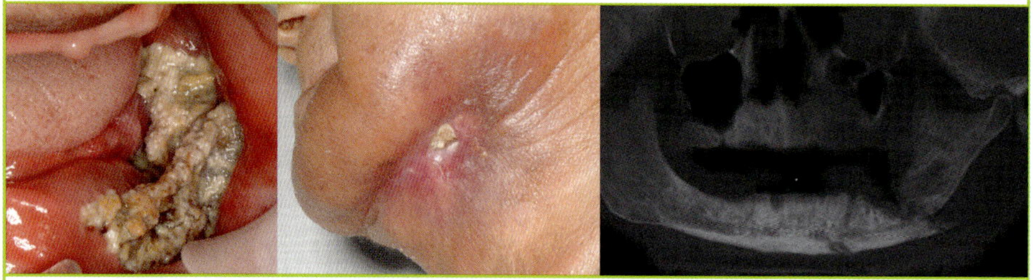

Patient evaluation

- **Chief complaint:** "The left side of my jaw is draining."
- **History of present illness:** This woman has known metastatic breast cancer for the past 6 years. She was treated with a radical mastectomy and chemotherapy of Faslodex and Ibrance as well as zoledronate 4 mg IV monthly for the past 3 years and 4 months (40 doses). Her last dose was last month. The reports from her oncologist that she brings with her indicate that her metastasis is stable and not advancing.
- **Previous medical history:** Atrial fibrillation, hypertension, no known drug allergies, hypercholesterolemia
- **Medications:** Eliquis (Bristol-Myers Squibb) 5 mg BID, amlodipine 5 mg/day, Lipitor, Ibrance
- **Oral examination:** There is a draining orocutaneous fistula at the left angle of the mandible. The mandible is mobile, implying a fracture at the left angle. The mandible is painful upon manipulation, and pus is expressed when manipulated. There is exposed, discolored brownish bone in the left alveolar process resembling an unhealed tooth socket. There are no other areas of exposed bone or masses noted. The mandible is deflected upon closing due to a malposition of the mandibular arch to the left from the pathologic fracture.
- **Radiographic examination:** There is a diffuse sclerosis in the mandibular angle area and an osteolysis to the inferior border with a slight separation consistent with a pathologic fracture. There are several splintered sequestra around the fracture.
- **Diagnosis:** Stage III DIONJ

Suggested course of action

1. Irrigate the fistula with 0.12% chlorhexidine and prescribe amoxicillin 500 mg TID ongoing and metronidazole 500 mg TID for a limit of 10 days.
2. Alert the oncologist as to your finding and plans for an inpatient surgery. Request a temporary discontinuation of the zoledronate (a drug holiday). →

Case 6 (cont)

3. Plan a surgery to resect the necrotic bone via a continuity resection from the midramus (vertical subcondylar type osteotomy) to an area 1 cm from the radiographically evident DIONJ. Consider a free vascular fibula reconstruction by scheduling a CT angiogram (CTA) to confirm the three-vessel runoff needed to safely harvest a fibula graft and plain films of each fibula to assess for metastatic deposits. Also consider an allogeneic nerve graft for the inferior alveolar nerve.
4. If the CTA identifies all three vessels to the leg below the knee and plain films rule out metastatic deposits in the fibula, proceed with the resection and free vascular fibula together with an allogeneic nerve graft for the best obtainable outcome.
5. If the CTA negates the use of a fibula or the plain films identify metastasis deposits in each fibula, then option for a 3-mm titanium plate reconstruction and a free fasciocutaneous flap (ie, radial forearm or anterior lateral thigh flap) if soft tissue replacement is required.

Rationale

- An infected pathologic fracture of DIONJ requires a resection for resolution. Although antibiotics may be useful in the short-term, the mobility around the fracture site will predictably allow a continuous ingress of bacteria for a persistent infection with symptoms.
- Many cases of continuity resection preclude bony reconstruction due to the involvement of donor bone. This is due to the possibility of malignant cells in the bone marrow of a cancellous marrow graft and the fact that rhBMP-2/ACS is contraindicated in patients with an active malignancy. However, this case illustrates a possible exception. Documenting a disease-free fibula together with the three vessels needed to ensure a safe fibula harvest allows for bony reconstruction.
- The bone graft will develop a bony union and recreate continuity of the mandible. In a young woman of 52 years, this will prevent the possibility of the plate loosening over time or a plate fracture. Due to the reduced sensitivity of the fibula to zoledronate, it may also accept dental implants to replace lost teeth if the oncologist continues the zoledronate drug holiday.

Case 7

A 63-year-old Hispanic woman with stable metastatic breast cancer presents with her daughter for Spanish translation.

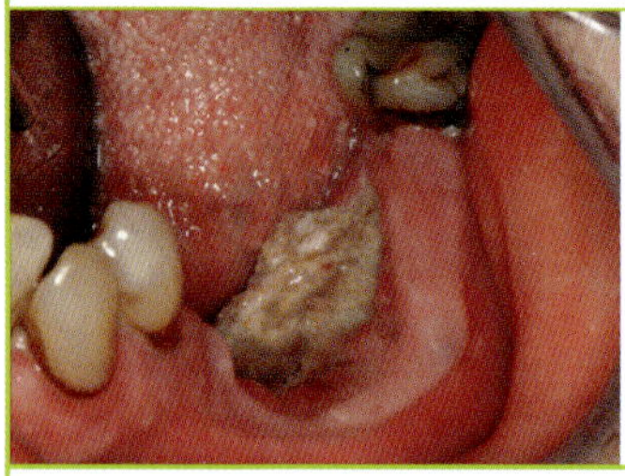

Patient evaluation

- **Chief complaint:** Pain and a swollen jaw on the left side
- **History of present illness:** Together, the patient and her daughter relate that the patient had been receiving zoledronate 4 mg IV for the past 2 years, which was well tolerated. However, when zoledronate was replaced by denosumab, she began to experience mobile teeth and exposed bone around teeth nos. 18, 19, and 20 after two doses of denosumab (once each month). Her dentist did not notice the exposed bone and removed the teeth under the diagnosis of "hopeless periodontitis." The patient has continued with pain and persistent swelling for the past 2 months resistant to clindamycin 300 mg three times daily. They relate that the area of exposed bone is increasing. Her oncologist stopped the denosumab 2 months ago.
- **Previous medical history:** Metastatic breast cancer, Hashimoto's thyroiditis, hypercholesterolemia, left breast lumpectomy. They report no known drug allergies.
- **Medications:** Faslodex, Synthroid, denosumab (discontinued 2 months ago)
- **Oral examination:** There is a 2.5-cm area of discolored brown exposed bone around the nonhealed sockets of teeth nos. 18, 19, and 20. The surrounding mucosa is edematous with a sight drainage. The left side of the face is also slightly swollen at the mandibular level as compared to the opposite side. There are no other areas of exposed bone. Tooth no. 21 is 1+ mobile. The remainder of the dentition is stable. The mandible is intact, and the sensation to the lower lip and chin is normal and equal bilaterally.
- **Radiographic examination:** A CBCT scan shows an osteolysis of the alveolar bone above the level of the mandibular canal and a marrow sclerosis below the level of the mandibular canal. There is also a developing involucrum and sequestration process of the lingual cortex extending as far anterior as the canine region. The mandibular canal is intact and completely within the sclerotic bone.
- **Diagnosis:** Stage I DIONJ

Suggested course of action

1. Discontinue the clindamycin and prescribe amoxicillin 500 mg three times daily ongoing and metronidazole 500 mg three times daily limited to 10 days. →

Case 7 (cont)

2. Alert the oncologist to your diagnosis and request a continued drug holiday from denosumab for another 2 months prior to a planned surgery followed by 3 months after surgery.
3. When the drug holiday reaches 4 months off of denosumab, proceed with an alveolectomy type surgery to remove all the necrotic bone above the mandibular canal. One should reflect the lingual mucosa to the midline area so as to also remove the sequestering lingual cortex. If available, place platelet-rich plasma (PRP) or a bone marrow aspirate into the resultant wound and gain a primary closure.
4. During surgery, IV amoxicillin 2 g and metronidazole 500 mg is recommended. Extend these medications orally for 7 days after surgery.

Rationale

- Clindamycin is not the best choice to control the secondary infection seen in DIONJ cases. This is because *Actinomyces* species are the most common microorganisms in DIONJ, to which clindamycin has limited sensitivity. Additionally, other common pathogens associated with DIONJ such as *Eikenella* and *Moraxella* are resistant to clindamycin.
- It is well known that the use of denosumab after a bisphosphonate often results in a rapid development of exposed bone and a severe expression of DIONJ. In this case, the 4-month drug holiday for denosumab reduces the complication potential from that drug due to its 26-day half-life. However, the drug holiday does not reduce the complication potential from the previous use of zoledronate due to its 11.2-year half-life. This risk is worthy to include in the informed consent.
- In the multicultural populations in most countries today, it is not uncommon to see patients that may not understand your discussion or treatment plan. It is advised to obtain adequate translation during the visit and document it. It is also necessary to include the name of the translator and their relationship to the patient in the consultation notes.
- It is somewhat characteristic that the lingual plate is involved at a distance from the clinically exposed bone. Therefore, it is prudent to also examine this area clinically and radiographically.
- The surgery must remove all the necrotic bone to bleeding, normal-appearing bone and round off all sharp edges. The fact that sclerotic bone is a margin does not indicate its removal. If the bone has good bleeding points despite its greater mineralization, it will heal.
- To gain a primary closure, one might need to score the periosteum and undermine the margin. The exposed bone by definition identifies a loss of soft tissue. Advancing the mucosa over the remaining viable bone and adding the progenitor cells and growth factors in PRP and/or a bone marrow aspirate from a radiographically uninvolved site will enhance the healing of the mucosa that has been compromised by chronic infection and a quantitative loss.

Case 8 A 47-year-old woman who is a fellow dentist

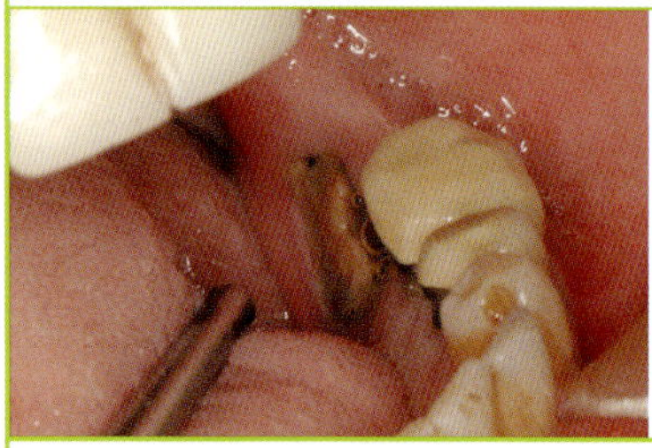

Patient evaluation

- **Chief complaint:** Exposed bone in the left lingual alveolar cortex around tooth no. 19. It has been present for 1 year and has not increased in size. It has been asymptomatic.
- **History of present illness:** She was diagnosed with multiple myeloma 5 years earlier and underwent a stem cell transplant with Revlimid and zoledronate therapy. She has been in remission for the past 2 years. A total-body PET scan 6 months ago showed no increase uptake, suggestive of multiple myeloma. Her zoledronate was discontinued 6 months ago when the exposed bone became evident.
- **Previous medical history:** An otherwise normal health history except for the multiple myeloma
- **Medications:** Only Revlimid currently. She reports no known drug allergies.
- **Oral examination:** There is a 1 cm area of white exposed bone opposite tooth no. 19. There is no drainage or edema. The exposed bone is nonmobile, but tooth no. 19 is 1+ mobile. An occlusal analysis identifies a high contact of the lingual cusp on tooth no. 14 onto tooth no. 19. The remainder of the oral examination shows no other areas of exposed bone, a balanced occlusion, and no other mobile teeth.
- **Radiographic examination:** A CBCT scan shows a slight demineralization around teeth nos. 19 and 20. However, the scan also shows several round radiolucent lesions in the right ramus. There are no other significant radiographic findings.
- **Diagnosis:** Stage I DIONJ: Possible reactivation of multiple myeloma

Suggested course of action

1. Alert the oncologist of your findings, focusing mostly on your film, particularly your suspicion of reactivated multiple myeloma. Send the oncologist a copy of your film.
2. Relieve the excessive occlusal contact between teeth nos. 19 and 14.
3. Consider splinting tooth no. 19 to nonmobile teeth anterior to it.
4. Prescribe a "pocket prescription" for amoxicillin 500 mg three times daily to be used if secondary infection develops.
5. Place the patient on a surveillance protocol every 3 months. →

Case 8 (cont)

Rationale

- The cancer for which a bisphosphonate or a RANK ligand inhibitor has been prescribed and which has caused DIONJ always has priority over the DIONJ. It is prudent to look for unexplained radiolucencies or masses in the jaws in such metastatic cancer patients that may reveal that the patient is out of remission.
- Although total-body PET scans are useful in detecting metastatic foci, they are not 100% sensitive for either metastatic cancer or DIONJ. That is, PET scans only identify areas of increased activity. Some cancer deposits will be static and not growing and therefore may not be recognized as an increased uptake. Similarly, an area of DIONJ that is dead bone with no vascularity will not show an increased uptake unless there is secondary infection or an inflammatory reaction to the exposed bone. In this case, neither DIONJ nor what turned out to be multiple myeloma punched-out lesions in the mandible were noted on the PET scan. A good panoramic film or a CBCT scan is actually a very good assessment for metastatic cancer to the jaws.
- Because this patient was asymptomatic and exhibited excellent plaque control, there was no indication to intervene with a debridement. The occlusal adjustment and splinting of teeth are intended to resist the progression of DIONJ in the face of a likely return to intensive multiple myeloma therapy. Therefore, a close surveillance of this patient is recommended.

Case 9 A 54-year-old man with controlled multiple myeloma

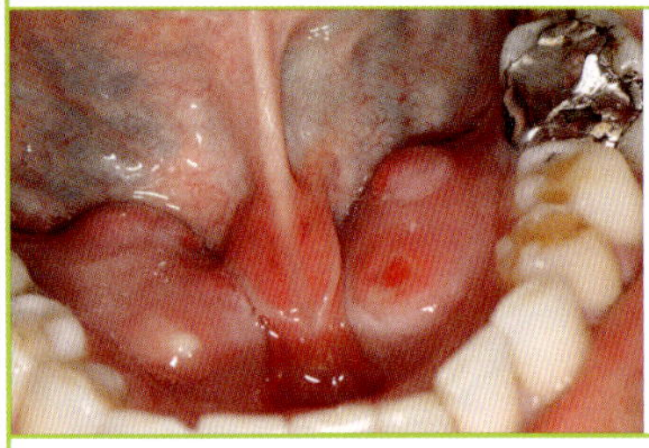

Patient evaluation

- **Chief complaint:** "I have exposed bone and pain" in the floor of the mouth.
- **History of present illness:** This man is currently on active treatment for multiple myeloma with Revlimid, cyclophosphamide, dexamethasone, and denosumab. He developed exposed bone over his lingual tori 6 months ago. It has been painful for the past 6 months, for which he has been prescribed oral Dilaudid (Fresenius Kabi), which he takes regularly. He relates that the Dilaudid is less effective than it was originally, so he supplements it with oxycodone 7.5 mg and marijuana. He relates that his pain is increasing. He received his last denosumab injection of 120 mg last week. He has not received any treatment for the exposed bone to date.
- **Previous medical history:** Multiple myeloma, hypertension, hypercholesterolemia. He reports no known drug allergies.
- **Medications:** Lopressor (Novartis), hydrochlorothiazide, rosuvastatin, denosumab, cyclophosphamide, dexamethasone
- **Oral examination:** There is exposure of two lingual tori in the floor of the mouth. The exposed tori are partially resorbed, creating jagged bone edges. The floor of the mouth is erythematous but not swollen. There is no drainage or fluctuation noted in the floor of the mouth or submental triangle.
- **Radiographic examination:** A CBCT scan shows osteolysis in each lingual torus. The osteolysis is limited to the tori and is not seen in other locations in either jaw.
- **Diagnosis:** *(1)* Stage II DIONJ because involved tori are on both sides of the midline (two quadrants). *(2)* Likely narcotic addiction.

Suggested course of action

1. Prescribe amoxicillin 500 mg three times daily ongoing and metronidazole 500 mg three times daily for the first 10 days as well as 0.12% chlorhexidine oral rinses.
2. Smooth jagged bone edges with an irrigated bur.
3. Alert the oncologist about the exposed bone and request a drug holiday of 4 months off the denosumab. Inform them that the other multiple myeloma drugs have little impact to this patient's DIONJ and can continue. Include your concerns about a narcotic addition and the expectation that the antibiotic regimen will reduce the pain level and the need for such combined analgesics. →

Case 9 (cont)

4. Offer addiction counseling and/or a pain center referral to the patient and inform him of the anticipated pain reduction with the compliant use of the prescribed antibiotics. Offer a prescription for hydrocodone 7.5 mg every 4 hours and/or ibuprofen 600 mg every 6 hours but not Dilaudid.
5. After the 4-month drug holiday, perform a bilateral torus excision and primary closure. It is useful to place PRP in the wound to enhance the healing but not a bone marrow aspirate in this case due to the multiple myeloma being a primary bone marrow malignancy. It may also be useful to place a lingual splint or a Coe-Pack to stabilize the repositioning of the lingual flap.
6. Be alert for narcotic withdrawal symptoms in the postoperative course.

Rationale

1. It is not uncommon for the pain of DIONJ to be sufficiently severe and relentless for a patient to develop a dependency on narcotic-based analgesics. Because the pain of DIONJ in most cases is due to secondary infection, the immediate prescriptions for the two most infection-controlling antibiotics is necessary. It is also recognized that sharp areas of exposed bone will frequently abrade the tongue, creating pain. Contouring the sharp edges will reduce this pain.
2. Restricting narcotic prescriptions while using antibiotic therapy avoids abuse.
3. Counseling the patient about a worsening narcotic dependence and alerting them to its risk is important. Offering addiction counseling is consistent with total patient care as well. In this case, a pain-management referral may also be advised because a drug holiday of 4 months is needed before a surgery that can resolve the DIONJ permanently and therefore the pain as well.

Case 10 A 67-year-old woman with metastatic breast cancer

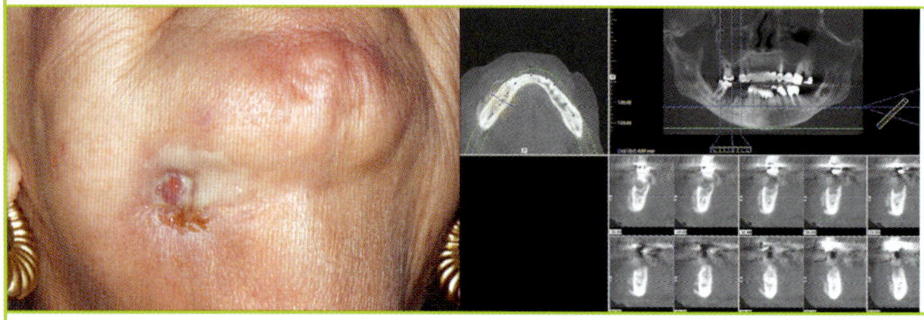

Patient evaluation

- **Chief complaint:** "I have an infection coming through my skin. It hurts and swells up periodically."
- **History of present illness:** Metastatic breast cancer for the past 6 years. The initial breast cancer 18 years ago was treated with a lumpectomy and chemotherapy. Metastasis to several vertebrae and scapula prompted intensive retreatment with multidrug chemotherapy including zoledronate. She received zoledronate 4 mg IV monthly for 5 years, but when exposed bone developed 1 year ago after mobile tooth no. 30 was removed, this regimen was changed to every 3 months. Her metastasis is under control with current therapy of Ibrance, Faslodex, and anastrozole. The zoledronate infusions have been withheld until your evaluation. The last infusion was 3 months ago.
- **Previous medical history:** Breast cancer with local surgery and chemotherapy, osteoporosis, no known allergies, allergic rhinitis
- **Medications:** Ibrance, Faslodex, anastrozole, and Zyrtec (Johnson & Johnson)
- **Oral examination:** There is an obvious orocutaneous fistula at the level of the inferior border in the molar region. It is draining a seropurulent discharge and has a diffuse edema of skin and of the oral mucosa. The area is painful to palpation. The mandible seems slightly expanded in the area. Orally, there is exposed bone in the unhealed socket of tooth no. 30 and part of the socket of tooth no. 29 as well. Tooth no. 31 has an exposed mesial root and shows signs of excessive wear. The maxillary dentition is heavily restored and has significant periodontal bone loss. However, there is no tooth mobility.
- **Radiographic examination:** A CBCT scan identifies the outline of unhealed tooth sockets nos. 29 and 30. Tooth no. 31 has a root canal treatment of both roots with apical radiolucencies. Both maxillary sinuses are opaque. The periodontal bone loss is noted to be moderate to severe in the maxillary molar region. Slices through the mandible show a diffuse deposition of extracortical bone as well as osteolysis in the central portion of the exposed bone.
- **Diagnosis:** Stage III DIONJ by virtue of osteolysis to the inferior border and an orocutaneous fistula →

Case 10 (cont)

Suggested course of action

1. Alert the oncologist of your diagnosis and request withholding zoledronate further in anticipation of surgery.
2. Prescribe amoxicillin 500 mg three times daily and metronidazole 500 mg three times daily for a 10-day limit in an effort to reduce secondary infection prior to a planned surgery.
3. Refer for a periodontal evaluation or accomplish limited scaling of the maxillary teeth along with 0.12% chlorhexidine irrigation as a temporary measure prior to mandibular surgery.
4. Accomplish a continuity resection of the right hemimandible with rigid titanium plate placement for continuity. **Note:** The patient declined microvascular fibula graft reconstruction due to concerns of metastases in many bones. During the 3 weeks between her initial examination and planned surgery, a second orocutaneous fistula developed, indicating the extent of the bony involvement to just short of the midline.
5. In a surgery of this nature, one must decide on the resection margins that will remove all of the necrotic bone and achieve maximum stability of the mandible. To lessen the chance of a return to surgery due to either residual DIONJ, a broken titanium plate, or a titanium plate that has become loose, one must plan for at least four bicortical locking screws in each residual segment and up to eight if healthy bone is available. As a guide to resection margins, the ramus does not contain alveolar bone, which is the most vulnerable bone for DIONJ. One should resect to bleeding bone in the ramus. The anterior resection margin is more problematic. For this margin, look for a resection edge that has viable bleeding bone marrow. If the patient has reactive extracortical bone as in this patient, that bone will be red in color and separate off the original cortex quite easily. Because that cortex is nonvital, the resection margin should be located in an area devoid of this extracortical reactive bone.

In many cases, such as this one, the titanium plate acting as an artificial jaw may represent the definitive reconstruction. Therefore, these plates should be 3-mm-thick reconstruction plates and placed with four or more bicortical locking screws on each end.

NOTE! Although this patient healed well with resolution of both fistulas, relief of pain, and alignment of her remaining occlusion, she developed exposed bone and an oral-antral fistula in the right maxilla 18 months later. This required removing the five teeth in the area, a complete sinus debridement, a buccal fat pad advancement, and a primary closure. This resolved the second focus of DIONJ and left her DIONJ-free with function limited to the opposite side. →

Case 10 (cont)

Rationale

- More than 5 years of regular zoledronate infusion results in a very high dose accumulation due to its 11.2-year half-life. It is not surprising and occurs on occasion that a second focus of DIONJ develops after resolution or control of a first focus. In this case, the inflammatory cytokines of uncontrolled periodontal disease causing an increase in bone remodeling was key to contributing to this emergence of a second DIONJ focus.
- The production of extracortical reactive bone underscores that the target of bisphosphonates and RANK ligand inhibitors is the osteoclast and that osteoclast death or dysfunction is the basic mechanism of DIONJ for these drugs. This is because the trabecular bone in the jaws is maintained by osteoclastic resorption and new bone formation by their release of growth factors. The periosteum develops bone independent of osteoclast bone resorption and growth factor release. The osteoblasts in the periosteum are not coupled to osteoclasts. They remain viable and form reactive bone in response to subperiosteal inflammation.
- The presentation with an orocutaneous fistula is indicative of advanced DIONJ and of significant secondary infection. Nonsurgical treatments or local debridements should not be expected to resolve this DIONJ presentation.

References

1. Marx RE. Oral and Intravenous Bisphosphonate-Induced Osteonecrosis of the Jaws: History, Etiology, Prevention, and Treatment, ed 2. Chicago: Quintessence, 2012:9–20.
2. Luckman SP, Hughes DE, Coxon FP, Graham R, Russell G, Rogers MJ. Nitrogen-containing bisphosphonates inhibit the mevalonate pathway and prevent post-translational prenylation of GTP-binding proteins, including Ras. J Bone Miner Res 1998;13:581–589.
3. Lacey DL, Boyle WJ, Simonet WS, et al. Bench to bedside: Elucidation of the OPG-RANK-RANKL pathway and the development of denosumab. Nat Rev Drug Discov 2012;11:401–419.
4. Gnant M, Pfeiler G, Steger GG, et al. Adjuvant denosumab in postmenopausal patients with hormone receptor-positive breast cancer (ABCSG-18): Disease-free survival results from a randomised, double-blind, placebo-controlled, phase 3 trial. Austrian Breast and Colorectal Cancer Study Group. Lancet Oncol 2019;20:339–351.
5. Cao Y, Langer R. A review of Judah Folkman's remarkable achievements in biomedicine. Proc Natl Acad Sci U S A 2008;105:13203–13205.
6. Folkman J. Angiogenesis: An organizing principle for drug discovery? Nat Rev Drug Discov 2007;6:273–286.
7. Barlesi F, Scherpereel A, Gorbunova V, et al. Maintenance bevacizumab-pemetrexed after first-line cisplatin-pemetrexed-bevacizumab for advanced nonsquamous nonsmall-cell lung cancer: Updated survival analysis of the AVAPERL (MO22089) randomized phase III trial. Ann Oncol 2014;25:1044–1052.
8. Ribatti D. From the discovery of vascular endothelial growth factor to the introduction of avastin clinical trials—An interview with Napoleone Ferrara. Int J Dev Biol 2011;55:383–388.
9. Zhou Q, Guo P, Gallo JM. Impact of angiogenesis inhibition by sunitinib on tumor distribution of temozolomide. Clin Cancer Res 2008;14:1540–1549.
10. Kollmannsberger C, Soulieres D, Wong R, Scalera A, Gaspo R, Bjarnason G. Sunitinib therapy for metastatic renal cell carcinoma: Recommendations for management of side effects. Can Urol Assoc J 2007;1(2 suppl):S41–S54.

Index

Page numbers followed by "t" denote tables; those followed by "f" denote figures.

A

Abaloparatide. *See* Recombinant human parathyroid hormone 1-80.
Abscesses, 42–43
Actinomyces, 32, 32f
Alendronate
  case studies involving, 40, 42
  DIONJ caused by, 3f, 4t, 30–31
  dosing of, 4, 4t, 6t
  drug holiday for, 40, 42, 53
  pamidronate versus, 60
  potency of, 3
  risk level for, 31
"All-on-4" concept, 44
Alveolar bone. *See also* Bone.
  biopsy of, 10, 11f
  osteoclast-mediated turnover of, 9
  remodeling and renewal of, 60
  surgical intrusion into, 10, 11f
Alveolectomy, 35
Amoxicillin, 33
Anastrozole, 23
Antiangiogenic drugs, 14–15, 16f, 59, 61
Antibiotics, 32–33
Antiosteoclastic drugs, 60–61
Apicoectomies, 28
Aromatase inhibitors
  definition of, 22
  osteopenia/osteoporosis induced by, 23

B

BAONJ. *See* Bisphosphonate-associated osteonecrosis of the jaws.
Bevacizumab, 14–15, 15f, 61, 66
Biopsy, alveolar bone, 10, 11f
Bisphosphonate(s). *See also* specific drug.
  complications of, 5
  denosumab after, 8, 8f, 81
  dose of, 4, 4t
  drug holidays from, 28–29
  duration of use, 7
  farnesyl synthase inhibition by, 60
  half-life of, 4
  osteoclast targeting by, 88
  potency of, 3, 4t
  route of administration, 7
Bisphosphonate-associated
  osteonecrosis of the jaws, 1
BMD. *See* Bone mineral density.
Bone. *See also* Alveolar bone.
  cellular composition of, 1
  remodeling of, 2, 8, 26f
  resorption of, 60
  turnover of, 2, 5, 8, 22
Bone mineral density, 21, 22f
Breast cancer, 68–69, 74–75, 80–81, 86–88
Bruxism, 64
Buccal fat pad
  blood supply of, 51
  reconstruction of, maxillary sinus
    debridement with, 35–36, 37f

C

Caldwell Luc approach, 35, 37f, 77
Cancer. *See also* Metastatic cancer.
  bone resorption associated with, 60
  breast, 68–69, 74–75, 80–81, 86–88
  case studies of, 68–88

DIONJ prevention and management in, 62–67, 63f, 65f
fractures from, 60
lung, 61, 76–77
osteoporosis patients versus, 59
prostate, 70–71
Candidiasis, 73
Caries, 64, 65
Case studies
breast cancer, 68–69, 74–75, 80–81, 86–88
cancer, 68–88
exposed bone, 72–73
lung cancer, 76–77
multiple myeloma, 72–73, 82–85
postmenopausal osteoporosis, 40–41, 46–47
postmenopausal women, 43–46, 48–55
teeth abscesses, 42–43
Checkpoint inhibitor, 77
Chemo-osteonecrosis of the jaws, 1
Chlorhexidine, 47, 55, 67
Chronic inflammation, 9
Clindamycin, 81
Comorbidities, 12
Computed tomography angiogram, 79
CONJ. *See* Chemo-osteonecrosis of the jaws.
Continuity resection of mandible, 36, 38, 39f, 79, 87
Corticosteroid-induced osteopenia/ osteoporosis, 23
Crown lengthening surgery, 10, 11f
C-terminal telopeptide test, 28–29, 43–46
CTX test. *See* C-terminal telopeptide test.
Cutaneous fistula, 25f, 49

D

Deep scaling, 63
Denosumab
after bisphosphonates, 8, 8f, 81
in cancer patients, 59
case study involving, 74–75
DIONJ caused by, 3f, 4t
dosing of, 4, 4t, 6t
drug holiday for, 29–30, 41, 67, 81, 84
half-life of, 4, 7, 75
mechanism of action, 5, 6f
osteoclasts affected by, 7
potency of, 3, 4t, 75
RANK ligand inhibition by, 6f, 61
risk level for, 31, 66
subcutaneous administration of, 7
Dental prophylaxis, 64
DEXA scan, 21
DIONJ. *See* Drug-induced osteonecrosis of the jaws.
Doxycycline, 32–33
Drug(s). *See also* specific drug.
antiangiogenic, 14–15, 16f, 59, 61
antiosteoclastic, 60–61
bisphosphonates. *See* Bisphosphonate(s).
dosing of, 4, 4t
half-life of, 4
length of time of use, 7
mechanism of action, 1–2, 5–7, 6t
potency of, 3
preventive measures before starting, 62–64
risk designation for, 31
route of administration, 7
Drug holidays
alendronate, 40, 42, 53
bisphosphonates, 28–29
case studies involving, 40–41, 47
denosumab, 29–30, 41, 67, 81, 84
effective use of, 28–30
pamidronate, 29
patient instruction regarding, 32
safety of, 30–31
for surgeries, 67
zoledronate, 29–30, 51, 65
Drug-induced osteonecrosis of the jaws
definition of, 12
management of. *See* Management.
prevention of, 62–67, 63f, 65f
risk factors for. *See* Risk factors.

staging of, 12–13, 13f–14f, 25f, 27f
terminology for, 1–2
Dual-energy x-ray absorptiometry scan, 21

E

Eikenella, 32
Etidronate, 3
Exposed bone, management of patients with
case study involving, 72–73
from DIONJ, 65–67
from osteopenia/osteoporosis drug, 31–39
Extraction sockets, 24, 25f
Extractions. *See* Tooth extractions.

F

Farnesyl synthase, 60
Femur fractures, 2, 3f, 21, 60
Fistula, 24f–25f, 78, 86
"Fragility fracture," 21, 22f

H

Hip joint, osteoporosis of, 22f
Hounsfield density, 21
Hypercalcemia, 60

I

Ibandronate, 31
dose of, 4, 4t
potency of, 3
Immune-based disease, drugs for, 16, 16f
Implants, 10, 11f, 79
Inflammation
chronic, 9
periodontal, 63
Initiating factors
chronic inflammation, 9
extractions, 8–9, 9t
surgical intrusion into alveolar bone, 10
traumatic occlusion, 9, 10f
Interleukin-6 inhibitor, 16
Involucrum, 26, 27f, 33, 34f, 55

L

Lamina dura sclerosis, 13f, 25, 25f, 69
Le Fort I osteotomy, 28
Letrozole, 23
Lingual cortex, mandibular
anatomy of, 26, 27f
posterior, 10, 12f, 24f
removal of, 34, 35f
Lung cancer, 61, 76–77

M

Management
antibiotics, 32–33
in cancer patients, 62–67, 63f, 65f
drug holidays, 28–31
nonsurgical, 31–33
of patients actively taking drugs known to cause DIONJ, 64–65
of patients with exposed bone
from DIONJ, 65–67
from osteopenia/osteoporosis drug, 31–39
of patients with no signs of DIONJ, 28–30
surgical, 33–39, 34f–39f
Mandible
continuity resection of, 36, 38, 39f, 79, 87
pathologic fracture of, 13, 14f, 27f
posterior lingual cortex of, 10, 12f
Mandibular sagittal split osteotomies, 28
Maxillary sinus
debridement of, with buccal fat pad reconstruction, 35–36, 37f
DIONJ involvement of, 13, 15f
floor of, 27f, 51
radiographic imaging of, 35, 37f
Maxillary sinusitis, 38f
Medicine-related osteonecrosis of the jaws, 1
Metastatic cancer
breast, 68–69, 74–75, 80–81, 86–88
prostate, 70–71

Methotrexate, 29
Metronidazole, 33, 67
Moraxella, 32
MRONJ. *See* Medicine-related osteonecrosis of the jaws.
Mucoceles, 35, 37f
Mucositis, chemotherapy-related, 64
Multiple myeloma, 72–73, 82–85

N

Necrotic bone
- *Actinomyces* colonies in, 32f
- exfoliation of, 33

Nivolumab, 77
Nonsurgical management, 31–33

O

Occlusal adjustments, 64
Occlusal balance, 65
Occlusal overloading, 47
Oral hygiene, 64–65
Oral-antral communication, 36, 37f
Oral-antral fistula, 87
Orocutaneous fistula, 86, 88
Orthodontics, 28
Osseocutaneous flap, 39f
Osteoblasts, 1
Osteoclasts
- bisphosphonate effects on, 60f
- cancer-stimulated, 60
- denosumab effects on, 7
- RANK ligand stimulation of, 2
- resorption by, 5f, 29f, 60
- zoledronate effects on, 69

Osteocytes, 1–2
Osteolysis, 26, 26f
Osteopenia
- aromatase inhibitor-induced, 23
- bisphosphonates for. *See* Bisphosphonates.
- definition of, 22f
- evaluation of, 23–27, 24f–27f
- oral examination in, 24, 24f–25f
- radiographic examination in, 25f–27f, 25–27
- steroid-induced, 23
- surgical management of, 33–39, 34f–39f

Osteoporosis
- aromatase inhibitor-induced, 23
- bisphosphonates for. *See* Bisphosphonates.
- bones susceptible to fractures, 21
- cancer patients versus, 59
- definition of, 21
- diagnosis of, 21
- evaluation of, 23–27, 24f–27f
- hip joint involvement, 22f
- oral examination in, 24, 24f–25f
- postmenopausal, 22–23, 40–41, 46–47
- radiographic examination in, 25f–27f, 25–27
- severe, 21, 53
- steroid-induced, 23
- surgical management of, 33–39, 34f–39f

Osteoprotegerin, 1
Osteosclerosis, 25, 26f

P

Pamidronate
- alendronate versus, 60
- dosing of, 60
- drug holidays for, 29
- risk level for, 62, 66
- zoledronate versus, 60

Pathologic fracture
- case study of, 78–79
- of mandible, 13, 14f, 27f

Penicillin, 33
Periodontal inflammation, 63
Periodontal osseous surgery, 10, 10f–11f, 28
Platelet-rich plasma, 34–35, 81
Poorly fitting appliances, 24, 25f
Posterior mandibular lingual cortex, 10, 12f, 24f
Postmenopausal osteoporosis, 22–23, 40–41, 46–47

Postmenopausal women, 43–46, 48–55
Prostate cancer, 70–71
PRP. *See* Platelet-rich plasma.

R

Radiographic examination, 25f–27f, 25–27
Raloxifene
  DIONJ caused by, 4t
  risk level for, 31
RANK ligand
  denosumab inhibition of, 6f, 61
  description of, 1–2, 5
  inhibition of, 5, 16, 41, 53, 88
  osteoclast secretion of, 60
Recombinant human bone morphogenetic protein-2/acellular collagen sponge, 38, 39f, 49, 52, 67, 79
Recombinant human parathyroid hormone 1-34
  DIONJ caused by, 4t
  risk level for, 31
  severe osteoporosis treated with, 53
Recombinant human parathyroid hormone 1-80
  DIONJ caused by, 4t
  risk level for, 31
Resorbing osteoclasts, 29f
rhBMP-2/ACS. *See* Recombinant human bone morphogenetic protein-2/acellular collagen sponge.
Risedronate
  DIONJ caused by, 4t
  dose of, 4, 4t
  potency of, 3
  risk level for, 31
Risk factors
  chronic inflammation, 9
  comorbidities, 12
  drugs, 3–8
  extractions, 8–9, 9t
  overview of, 2–3
  periodontal osseous surgery, 10, 10f–11f, 28
  torus, 10–11, 12f
  traumatic occlusion, 9, 10f
  vulnerable sites, 10–11, 12f
Root banking, 65f

S

Scaling, deep, 63
Sequestrectomy, 32, 34, 54
Splint therapy, 64–65
Staging, 12–13, 13f–14f, 25f, 27f
Steroid-induced osteopenia/osteoporosis, 23
Sunitinib, 15, 16f, 61, 66

T

Teeth abscesses, 42–43
Teriparatide. *See* Recombinant human parathyroid hormone 1-34.
Third molars, partial bony impacted, 63, 63f
Tiludronate, 3
Titanium reconstruction plate, 39f
Tocilizumab, 16, 16f
Tooth extractions
  description of, 8–9, 9t
  nonrestorable teeth, 63, 63f
  sockets from, 24, 25f
  third molars, 63f
Tooth mobility, 24, 25f, 65
Torus, 10–11, 12f, 24, 25f, 54
Trabecular bone, 26, 26f
Traumatic occlusion, 9, 10f
T-score, 21, 22f
Tyrosine kinase inhibitors, 15

V

Vascular endothelial growth factor, 14, 49, 61
VEGF. *See* Vascular endothelial growth factor.
Veillonella, 32
Vitamin D3, 31

Z

Zithromycin, 33
Zoledronate
DIONJ caused by, 7, 8f, 50
dosing of, 6t, 30
drug holidays for, 29–30, 51, 65
half-life of, 65, 81, 88
osteoclastic bone remodeling and renewal affected by, 69
pamidronate versus, 60
risk level for, 31, 62, 66
route of administration, 7